Contents

Acknowledgements

We are grateful to the Research and Development Division of the Department of Health for financing this research and for the help and advice we have received from Dr Ruth Chadwick.

From the start of the project, we benefited from the constructive comments of all the members of the Advisory Group: Professors Anthony Mann and Bob Woods (joint chairs), John Allcock, Dr Ruth Chadwick, Naomi Connelly, Briony Enser, Laura Kline, Helen Krizka, Val Manchee, Dr Ann Netten, Danny Palnoch and David Ward. We should also like to thank the anonymous referees who have commented on earlier drafts.

We thank all our colleagues in the Research Unit for their willing contributions. In particular, we should like to thank the Director Professor Mike Fisher, the former Director Professor Jan Pahl, Senior Research Fellow Enid Levin, the Unit Administrator Rose Freeman and the Unit Secretary Veronica Barker. We owe particular debts of thanks to Toby Andrew for his statistical advice and to Linda Dolan who entered much of the data. We should also like to thank Ann Netten, Angela Hallam and Jane Knight of the PSSRU for working on the costings and writing Chapter 8.

We are grateful to our dedicated team of interviewers: Jan Brownfoot, Marian Buxton, Diane Fletcher, Christine Furmston, Samantha Goldberg, Rosemary Lawrance, Beryl Riley, Chloé Rowlings and Jean Smith.

We appreciate all the assistance we received from all the staff in the social services departments in which we worked, in particular the social workers and administrative staff, who went to considerable lengths to help us. Above all, we must thank all the older people, carers and proxy informants for setting aside so much time to share their thoughts and experiences with us.

List of tables and figures

Tables

Figures

Glossary and abbreviations

AA/DLA	Attendance Allowance Disability Living Allowance: benefit paid to people who need help with personal care because of illness or disability.
ADL	Activities of Daily Living. In this study they were defined as transfer, washing, bathing, dressing, using the lavatory, eating, rising and retiring, self-medicating and leaving the house (10 items) (Levin et al, 1989).
ADS	Alzheimer's Disease Society (now Alzheimer's Society)
ADSS	Association of Directors of Social Services
assessment	Unless specifically mentioned in the text, 'assessment' refers to assessments completed under Section 47 of the 1990 National Health Service (NHS) and Community Care Act.
average	Tables specify whether the mean or median is used. For ease of reading the term 'average' is used in the text, except in Chapter 8 where 'mean', and 'median' are used.
BAS	Brief Assessment Schedule (Macdonald et al, 1982): an interview schedule designed to screen for dementia and depression. It comprises two scales:
	(i) the Organic Brain Scale (OBS), to test the presence and severity of dementia. Scores range from 0 to 8 and are divided as follows: no dementia (0-2); mild to moderate dementia (3-7); severe dementia (8);
	(ii) the Depression Scale (DEP). Scores range from 0 to 24. The cut-off point for symptoms consistent with a depressive illness is 7.
BVPI	Best Value Performance Indicator
carer	Always refers to non-professional care given by family member or friend. Carers who live with the person for whom they care are described as 'co-resident carers'; those who do not are described as 'non-resident' carers.
CL	confidence limit
CPN	community psychiatric nurse
DEP	See BAS.
DoH	Department of Health
DHSS	Department of Health and Social Security

DSM	*Diagnostic and Statistical Manual of Mental Disorders.* The terms DSM III, DSM III R and DSM IV denote the edition of the manual that was used.
DSS	Department of Social Security
day care	Includes both day centres and NHS day hospitals. There were isolated examples of attendance at day clubs.
GHQ-28	Self-completion questionnaire administered to carers. Scores over 6 are taken to indicate 'caseness' for symptoms usually associated with depression, anxiety or hypochondriacal self-concern.
GHS	General Household Survey, a continuous survey of a random sample of the general population living in private households.
GP	general practitioner
home care	Care provided in the home by local authority and private agencies where the emphasis is on assistance with personal care and household tasks.
home-based carer support	Care provided in the home in which the emphasis is on providing the person with dementia with opportunities for social engagement at the same time as giving carers a break.
IADLs	Instrumental Activities of Daily Living. In this study they were defined as shopping, housework, food preparation, laundry, household maintenance and managing money (six items) (Levin et al, 1989).
ICA	Invalid Care Allowance: benefit paid to people aged 16-65 who spend at least 35 hours a week caring for a severely disabled person who is in receipt of AA or DLA. An earnings limit operates for the receipt of this benefit.
living in the community	Refers to people living in private households, including sheltered accommodation. Used synonymously with 'at home' in this report.
LA	local authority
LTC	Long-term care: refers to care in residential or nursing homes or NHS continuing care.
NHS	National Health Service
NISW	National Institute for Social Work
NISW Noticeable Problems	Six-item informant questionnaire designed to screen for cognitive impairment (see Levin et al, 1989).
OBS	See BAS.
ONS	Office for National Statistics; formerly the Office of Population, Censuses and Surveys (OPCS)
OT	occupational therapist
PSSRU	Personal Social Services Research Unit
proxy informant	Usually refers to a paid member of staff involved in the care of the older person. Non-professionals were divided into proxy or carer informants on the basis of the frequency and type of care they gave to the older person. There were only three non-professional proxy informants (one neighbour and two family friends).
referral	Other than in Chapter 2, when we use the term 'referral', it signifies a referral that resulted in an assessment (qv).

short-term breaks	Refers to stays by the older person of 24 hours or more in a residential, nursing home, NHS hospital or adult placement scheme. Overnight care provided in the home was included under home-based carer support (qv).
significance	A p value of 0.05 means that the observed result has a 5% (1 in 20) probability of occurring by chance. A p value of 0.01 means that the observed result has a 1% (1 in 100) probability of occurring, and a p value of 0.001 means a probability of 0.1%. The value $p = 0.05$ is conventionally used as the threshold of significance, with a value below 0.05 being considered significant. (In other words, the event is unlikely to have occurred by chance and therefore warrants an explanation.)
social worker	We use the term 'social worker' in favour of any other term such as 'care manager' because it is the term that most study participants appear to know and understand and because most of the assessments were completed by qualified social workers.
social work interview	Research interview with assessor, almost always a social worker.
SD	standard deviation
SSD	Social Services Department
SSI	Social Services Inspectorate
SWSG	Scottish Office Social Work Services Group
Time One	Study stage occurring approximately six months after the older person's referral to the SSD during which interviews were completed with carers, older people and proxy informants.
Time Two	Study stage occurring approximately 18 months after the older person's referral to the SSD during which interviews were completed with carers, older people and proxy informants.

Introduction

Key points

- This chapter outlines the context for the community care changes and discusses the key literature on services for people with dementia.

- People with dementia are major users of long-term care and community services.

- The community care changes have highlighted the need for a study focusing on the approach that social services departments (SSDs) were taking towards care for people with dementia.

- Different frameworks for evaluating services for people with dementia are described, including costs of care, patterns of service use, entry rates to long-term care, the role of specialist schemes, support for carers and user views.

- Messages from existing research highlight the considerable costs of dementia care in terms of community and long-term care, variation in service provision throughout the country, inconsistent impacts on entry rates to long-term care from the provision of intensive specialist services, and the risk of poor psychological health among carers of people with dementia. The views of people with dementia who are service users are under-represented.

It is arguable that the White Paper Caring for people (1989) and the subsequent National Health Service and Community Care Act 1990 constituted the first significant attempt to introduce a coherent legislative framework and a planned programme of implementation which not only married financial and organisational arrangements with a number of key political objectives but also embraced all groups of adult service users and carers. (Hughes, 1995, p 1)

Study scope

This book is an account of a study that was based on a sample of people with dementia who were referred to three social services departments (SSDs) between November 1994 and February 1995 and who went on to receive an assessment. They were followed up over an 18-month period.

The research was commissioned by the Department of Health (DoH) as part of a wider programme designed to monitor the effects of the 1990 National Health Service (NHS) and Community Care Act. It was commissioned after the Act was implemented and so is not a 'before and after' study through which the new system and its predecessor might be compared directly. The programme also included studies of care management (Challis, 1994; Challis et al, 1998), an evaluation of community care for elderly people (ECCEP Team, 1998) and the experiences of social work practitioners and managers (Levin and Webb, 1997).

Overall, the published research literature that is based on data collected after April 1993, when the 1990 National Health Service (NHS) and Community Care Act was fully implemented, is relatively small. Research activity has tended to concentrate on management processes and strategic change. Hence the experiences of local authorities in the aftermath of the community care changes have been comprehensively described by Lewis and Glennerster (1996) and Lewis (1997). In addition to the studies that were mentioned earlier (Challis, 1994; Challis et al, 1998), published accounts of care management in England include the Department of Health (DoH) (1994), Social Services Inspectorate (SSI) (1998a), and in Scotland (Petch et al, 1996). There is less published work on the experiences of users and carers and practitioners. The views of older users have been considered by MacDonald (1999), and the experiences of users and practitioners during the interval between the passing of the legislation and its final implementation have been documented by Caldock (1992a, 1992b, 1992c). Information from the ECCEP study (Davies and Fernandez, in press) which replicates work completed before the community care changes (Davies et al, 1990) will provide the best source of information on how the system serving older people post-April 1993 compares with its predecessor.

The comparative shortage of published research has meant that much of the current evidence on the effect of the community care changes has been derived from SSI inspections, small-scale projects and internal monitoring (Parker, 1998). This lends additional importance to studies such as this one, which have an evaluative design. Its focus on the direct experiences of people with dementia and their carers accords with the tradition of previous work in the National Institute for Social Work (NISW) Research Unit (Levin et al, 1989, 1994).

Background to the community care changes

A commitment to the concept of community care can be identified from the earliest years of the postwar welfare state. During the 1950s and 1960s, the phrase appeared with increasing frequency in official reports and politicians' speeches (Walker,

1995). Community care initiatives in the 1970s concentrated mainly on influencing the degree of coordination between health and social care through planning processes, financial transfers and financial incentives (Webb and Wistow, 1986). However, a change occurred in the early 1980s, when the Department of Health and Social Security (DHSS) undertook a series of studies on health and social services. The study on community care examined the extent to which there had been a shift in the balance of care from long-term institutional care to other forms of provision. Emphasis was also laid on the role of the voluntary sector and carers (DHSS, 1981). This began a move away from focusing on organisational structures and towards examining outcomes for individual clients (Challis et al, 1995).

By the end of the 1980s existing policy was coming under increasing scrutiny. Three factors in particular appear to have contributed to the situation (Henwood, 1992). The first was a response to studies completed in the 1970s which looked at the changing age structure of the population. At the time, predictions tended to take an extremely pessimistic view both about the numbers of people requiring care and about the numbers of family members who would be available to provide it. The second was the realisation that official policy objectives did not always reflect the realities of care 'on the ground'. For instance, the extent to which schemes to close long-stay geriatric and psychogeriatric beds during the 1980s had been matched by an expansion of services for older people living in the community was felt to be limited (Sinclair et al, 1990). The third was the emergence of the 'new managerialism' (Davies, 1987), an approach exemplified in an influential Audit Commission report (1986) which had pointed out that fragmented responsibilities for implementing policies between health and social services often resulted in duplication and gaps in service provision.

Such concerns were given an added urgency by the effect of changes in 1980 to the rules under which people could claim board and lodging expenses from the Department of Social Security (DSS). Under this arrangement, the fees of older people who could not afford to pay for their own residential and nursing home care could be reimbursed up to a local set limit, enabling people to select a home personally, rather than having to apply to the local authority or wait for a vacancy in an NHS long-stay bed. This acted as a 'perverse incentive' so that, despite the official policy objectives in favour of developing services to enable people to remain in their own homes, there was a rapid increase in residential and nursing home places in the independent sector that was not commensurate with the growth in the number of people aged 75 and over. The effect was to increase this part of the DSS budget from £10 million in 1979 to over £2,000 million in 1991 (Lewis and Glennerster, 1996).

The political sequelæ are well known. Following his earlier report on the management of the NHS, Sir Roy Griffiths was asked to inquire into the way in which public funds were used to support community care policy and to advise on options for improvement. His main proposals – (a) that public finance should be provided only following separate assessments of the financial needs of applicants and of their needs for care; (b) that this should be managed by local authority SSDs; and (c) that steps should be taken to encourage the development of the private and voluntary sectors in order to create a 'mixed economy of care' (DoH, 1988) – were accepted in the White Paper *Caring for people* (Secretaries of State for Health, Social Security, Wales and Scotland, 1989). Subsequent legislation in the form of the 1990 NHS and Community Care Act gave SSDs the role as lead agency responsible for providing, or arranging to provide, community care services and responsibility for assessing individuals' needs for such services.

Historically, the term 'community care' had been used to convey a wide range of policy goals that were often conflicting (Lewis and Glennerster, 1996). *Caring for people* defined it as the:

> *... means [of] providing the services and support which people who are affected by problems of ageing, mental illness, mental handicap or physical or sensory disability need to be able to live as independently as possible in their own homes, or in homely settings in the community.* (Secretaries of State for Health, Social Security, Wales and Scotland, 1989, p 3)

Among the objectives of the changes were to:

> *... promote the development of domiciliary, day, and respite services to enable people to live in their own homes wherever feasible and sensible ... to ensure that service providers make practical support for carers a high priority [and] ... to make proper assessment of need and good case management the cornerstone of high quality care.* (Secretaries of State for Health, Social Security, Wales and Scotland, 1989, p 5)

Case management was later renamed care management. Originally a North American concept, the evidence for its adoption in the United Kingdom comes from the results of a series of studies completed by the Personal Social Services Research Unit (PSSRU) (Challis et al, 1987, 1995; Davies and Challis, 1986; Davies et al, 1990). Models of care management vary according to the client group for whom it is provided, but their functions are usually identified as the coordination of care arrangements to create a comprehensive response to need (Challis et al, 1995). The SSI/ Scottish Office Social Work Services Group (SWSG) defined the seven core tasks of care management as: publishing information, determining the level of assessment, assessing need, care planning, implementing the care plan, monitoring, and reviewing (SSI/SWSG, 1991a).

At the same time, the community care changes can also be seen as reflecting a wider trend within Europe, North America and Australia:

> *These patterns of change are designed to produce ... degree of downward substitution in the provision of care, moving away from institutional care, towards enhanced home care, and developing improved co-ordination at the client level.* (Challis, 1992, p 773)

They also reflected greater recognition for the contribution made by carers. In April 1996, the implementation of the 1995 Carers (Recognition & Services) Act meant that carers providing, or intending to provide, 'a substantial amount of care on a regular basis' could ask that their 'abilities to provide and to continue to provide care' also be assessed when the person for whom they cared was assessed under the 1990 NHS and Community Care Act.

Why focus on community care for people with dementia?

It is not difficult to perceive care for [people with dementia] as representing one of the greatest challenges to the development of welfare services throughout the western world. (Gilleard, 1992, p 310)

The service users who gave [social services] departments the greatest difficulty and cause for concern were – for all types of authority – elderly people suffering from mental infirmity or dementia and especially those presenting challenging behaviour. (ADSS, 1994, p 4)

The above quotations suggest the importance, but also the challenges, that are inherent in achieving successful community care for people with dementia. The remainder of this chapter discusses why it was important to examine their use of community and long-term care services in the context of the community care changes.

What is dementia?

The term 'dementia' is used to cover a range of progressive disorders that are characterised by a decline in intellectual and cognitive functioning. The most common type of dementia is Alzheimer's Disease, which is believed to affect around 60% of those people with dementia. Vascular dementia and dementia of the Lewy body type are generally reported to be the next most common, in that order, although some reviews have suggested that the former may be over-diagnosed and the latter under-diagnosed (Amar and Wilcox, 1996). Depending upon the type of dementia that he or she has, an individual will be affected in various ways. However, the main diagnostic criteria are that the ability to learn new information or recall previously learned information is affected, and that there are other disturbances, such as difficulties in language (aphasia), recognising objects or people (agnosia), completing motor activities such as dressing (apraxia), and in more complicated areas, such as abstract thinking or following a sequence of tasks. Personality and behavioural changes may also occur. The deficits must represent a decline from a previous level of ability and be severe enough to cause significant impairment in social and occupational functioning. Diagnoses are made after

excluding other potential causes, such as physical illnesses (American Psychiatric Association, 1994).

Although the precise reasons why people develop dementia remain uncertain, there have been major advances in our understanding of the factors increasing an individual's risk of being affected. The development of Alzheimer's Disease in later life (as happens in the majority of cases), has been linked with possession of the apolipoprotein E gene. A study has suggested that there is an interaction between apolipoprotein E and atherosclerosis in the aetiology of Alzheimer's Disease (Hofman et al, 1997).

Smaller numbers of people have a familial form of the disease. Environmental factors, such as head trauma, are also thought to play a role in some cases. While it is likely that applications for licences for new forms of drug treatment will be made in the future, the only treatments currently licensed in the UK for people with mild and moderate Alzheimer's Disease are donezepil (Aricept) and rivastigmine (Exelon). These drugs operate by blocking the enzyme that attacks the chemical acetycholine which is involved in the areas of the brain that control learning and memory and which are gradually destroyed as the disease advances. While unable to prevent these changes, the drugs are thought to slow the rate at which they occur.

Prevalence

The frequency of dementia rises with age. There is a doubling of the prevalence rate with every five-year increase from the age of 60 up to 95 years of age. Hofman and colleagues (1991) pooled and re-analysed data on the prevalence of dementia from 12 European studies. They included only studies in which all subjects had been personally examined using DSM III or equivalent criteria, because differences in assessment techniques and the criteria for making a diagnosis or rating the severity of dementia can influence the reported prevalence rates between studies (O'Connor et al, 1989a). Similarly, prevalence rates among people living in the community will be influenced by the supply and availability of long-term care locally (Gilleard, 1992), and so their analysis consisted of studies that included both people in the community and those in long-term care. It has been described as the most satisfactory recent compilation of prevalence data (Melzer et al, 1994). They concluded that the overall prevalence rates were 1.4% in the 64-69 year age group, rising to 13.0% in the 80-84 age group and 21.6% in the 85-89 age group. Among those aged under 75, the prevalence of dementia was slightly higher in men than women; in those aged 75 years or over, the prevalence was higher in women (Hofman et al, 1991).

In the UK, it has been estimated that the number of people with dementia is likely to grow from the present 650,000 to 855,000 by the year 2020 (DoH, 1997). This is mainly attributable to demographic changes that have led to an increase in the number of people aged 85 and over. The high prevalence rates in this age group mean that the predicted increase in the number of people with moderate and severe cognitive impairment will outpace the overall growth in the older population (Melzer et al, 1997).

Although only a minority of older people develop dementia, it must still be regarded as a major challenge for health and social care. This is because of its severe consequences for the lives of those who are affected and for their families.

Costs of dementia care

The projected increase in the numbers of people with dementia make it likely that the overall costs of care for this group will rise in the future (Wimo et al, 1997). A high proportion of current expenditure on nursing and residential care (Gray and Fenn, 1993), and on community services in the form of home care, meals services and attendance at day centres (Livingston et al, 1997), is already spent on supporting people with dementia. It has been estimated that in 1992/93 the direct costs of dementia to health and social services amounted to £850 million, the equivalent of 3.2% of all attributable public health and social services expenditure, excluding SSD children's services (Knapp et al, 1998). This figure does not include the direct costs borne by carers. These cover assistance in the form of financial support to the person with dementia by the carer or the cost of travelling to his or her home. Neither does it

comprise carers' indirect costs. These are harder to measure because opinions vary as to how they should be calculated. One method involves calculating the costs of replacing carers' time with paid care. Another considers carers' opportunity costs, such as giving up paid employment or loss of personal time. There are also caring impact costs in the form of increased use of healthcare services caused by carer depression or ill-health (Knapp et al, 1998). Chapter 8 explains the principles and methods by which the costs of packages of care for people with dementia might be calculated.

Use of long-term care and community services by people with dementia

People with dementia are at increased risk of entry into long-term care (Opit and Pahl, 1993). Overall, it has been estimated that almost half of all those living in all forms of institutional care have diagnostic levels of cognitive impairment (MRC CFAS and RIS, 1999). However, variation in the proportion of residents with dementia will vary between homes. Two studies, one pre-April 1993 (Ashby et al, 1989) and one post-April 1993 (Schneider et al, 1997a), reported prevalence rates of 78% and 79% respectively in the residential homes under examination. Another post-April 1993 study screened 308 people newly admitted to residential and nursing care using the Mini Mental State Examination (MMSE) (Folstein et al, 1975); almost two thirds had scores of 17 or under, a threshold generally taken to denote severe cognitive impairment (Mozley et al, 1999).

Currently 36% of older people with moderate or severe cognitive impairment are estimated to be living in long-term care. A further 36% need constant care or supervision but are living in the community supported chiefly by their spouses or children (Melzer et al, 1997, p 462).

There are few estimates available of the proportion of people with dementia living in the community who are in touch with health and social services. Using a multi-service census, Gordon and colleagues (1997) estimated that about half the people with dementia living in the community in

Tayside were known to either community health services, the social work department or voluntary organisations. A community survey of all older people living in an electoral ward in North London found that 60% had been in contact with some form of service in the previous month and that people with dementia were likely to be using more than one service (Cullen et al, 1993). In Cambridge, 51% of people with mild dementia received one or more of the following: home care, meals, day care or district nursing, either singly or in combination. This proportion rose to 62% of people with moderate dementia and 76% of people with severe dementia. By comparison, only 21% of the people without dementia received any of these services (O'Connor et al, 1989b).

The section on prevalence mentioned that the proportion of people with dementia using community services locally would be influenced by how much and what type of long-term care was available. Screening *across* community and long-term settings involves higher numbers and is likely to be more complex logistically. This may explain why, with a few exceptions (Macdonald et al, 1982; MRC CFAS and RIS MRC CFAS, 1999), studies of service use rarely include both community and long-term care residents.

The literature on service use has also identified issues in the way services are currently provided that would appear to give cause for concern.

Underprovision

Dementia has been shown to be associated with a high level of unmet need, mainly for more mainstream support and help with supervision (Philp et al, 1995).

Variation in provision

People with similar needs living in different parts of the country can receive different types of services (Burholt et al, 1997).

Inequalities in service allocation between groups with similar needs

Re-analysis of the Cambridge data set showed that cognitively impaired older women received less help from meals, home care and community nursing services than their counterparts with physical disabilities who were living in similar circumstances (Ely et al, 1997).

Differential service use by people from minority ethnic groups

A community survey in Liverpool found that people from minority ethnic communities with dementia or with depression were under-represented across health and social services and voluntary organisations. Interviews suggested that they were either unaware of the existence of services or believed them to be culturally inappropriate (Boneham et al, 1997).

The role of specialist community care services for people with dementia

Three studies have looked at the impact of specialist community services in enabling people with dementia to remain at home. A study looking at the impact of two home support schemes compared with two groups receiving 'standard provision' found that, while praised by the clients and their families, the schemes did not result in delayed entry to long-term care, improved well being, or self-care capacity in the people with dementia. However, the results were thought to have been influenced by the small sample size, and it was suggested that they did seem to be more effective than standard provision for people with severe dementia without family carers who did not need high levels of supervision (Askham and Thompson, 1990). O'Connor and colleagues (1991) found that an early intervention service giving access to a wide range of services for people living in the north of Cambridge did not affect admission rates to long-term care when compared with a group of similar people living in the south of the city. The authors concluded that the results may have been influenced by the timing of the evaluation (it took place at an early stage in the team's existence) and suggested that the intervention team might have identified people at potential risk earlier.

Challis and colleagues (1997) matched 43 individuals living in Lewisham, who had been assessed by a specialist multidisciplinary team and who went on to receive care management, with 43 people under the care of a similar team but without a care management service. After two years, 51% of the 'experimental' group were still at home, compared with 33% of the 'controls'. In Lewisham, members of both groups were supported by specialist multidisciplinary teams, as were members of the experimental group in Cambridge. However, the experimental group in Lewisham was also supported by care managers. In addition, unlike Cambridge, where the suitability of traditional home help and meals services for people with dementia and their carers was questioned (O'Connor et al, 1989b), the care managers in Lewisham were able to combine their specialist mental health support role with the ability to arrange for the provision of intensive care in the home. Challis et al (1997) concluded that it was this focus on both service structure and content that contributed to the positive outcomes for the experimental group.

Evaluating the effectiveness of services for people with dementia

Most people receiving community and long-term care services have a long-term illness or disability. The services they receive tend to be aimed at *maintaining* rather than *improving* their condition (Qureshi et al, 1998). Since service receipt is unlikely to result in dramatic improvements in functioning for people with dementia, great reliance has been placed on using entry rates to long-term care as a means of evaluating the effectiveness of community services. However, some researchers have challenged their suitability as an outcome measure. First, an overall reduction in the number of people with dementia admitted to long-term care may not be achievable in view of their increased risk of entry to residential and nursing homes (Ramsay et al, 1995). Second, measuring changes in service gives no indication of their ultimate effect on users and carers (Qureshi et al, 1998).

Supporting carers

One of the most striking developments that has occurred in recent years is the increased recognition of the contribution made by carers and other family members. The literature on caring is now substantial. Much of the early work examined caring from a gender perspective, as part of women's unpaid work (Finch and Groves, 1983; Ungerson, 1987; Dalley, 1988; Lewis and Meredith, 1988). Secondary analysis of the 1985 General Household Survey (GHS) (Green, 1988) suggested that gender was a less important factor than kinship tie in so far as co-resident carers (those who live with the person for whom they care) were concerned. It is widely recognised that ageist assumptions about older people as care receivers may lead to an under-recognition of their role as caregivers; where the person receiving help has a spouse, it is the spouse who is likely to be providing considerable amounts of care (Arber and Ginn, 1991). The issue of different levels of involvement has also been examined. The findings of Parker and Lawton (1994) confirmed support for the viewpoint that, while the provision of practical help in the form of shopping or gardening is the sort of activity that might be carried out by neighbours or distant family members, by contrast, help with intimate personal care tasks is almost always restricted to close family members (Qureshi and Walker, 1989; Wenger, 1992). To convey these distinctions, Parker and Lawton suggested distinguishing between 'heavily involved carers' and 'helpers'.

There are many ways in which caring has been demonstrated to have an impact. Many carers give considerable amounts of personal care, often while in poor health themselves. Carers who no longer have time to meet up with family members and friends, or to pursue hobbies and other leisure activities, may report feeling socially isolated and lonely. If they *are* given time off through the provision of respite services or help from other family members, much of it may have to be spent undertaking household tasks such as shopping or cleaning which they would otherwise be unable to do (Levin et al, 1994). Relationships between carers and those for whom they care may alter. Those who have never felt close to the person for whom they care, or who do so no longer, may be more inclined to relinquish caring (Hinrichsen and

Niederehe, 1994). Caring commitments may result in people forgoing promotion prospects, working part-time or retiring early. This may have long-term repercussions. For instance, women are especially vulnerable to financial disadvantage in old age if their work history has made it harder for them to acquire a personal or occupational pension (Ginn and Arber, 1996). It is important to recognise that the effects outlined above not only occur while a person is caring, but are likely to persist once the caring has ceased. They are what McLaughlin and Ritchie (1994) call the 'legacies of caring'.

At the same time, there is now much more pressure to move from generalised assumptions about caring towards theoretical approaches that more clearly reflect the complexities of caring relationships. We need an appreciation of the positive feelings that may be experienced (Grant and Nolan, 1993), and of continued reciprocities that blur distinctions between 'carer' and 'cared for'. It has been suggested that more work is required on developing an understanding of the circumstances in which men care (Fisher, 1994).

The importance of the role played by carers of people with dementia makes it essential that service evaluations are also able to consider outcomes for carers (Higginson et al, 1997). Ways of evaluating the effects of services on carers have been reviewed by Bourgeois and colleagues (1996), Morris and colleagues (1988), Teri (1999) and Woods (1992).

Two studies based on random community samples of carers have suggested that carers of people with dementia may be at greater risk of psychological ill-health than other carers (Livingston et al, 1996; Buck et al, 1997). A third (Eagles et al, 1987), suggested that such carers did not have higher levels of psychological ill-health but did have significantly raised levels of stress.

In non-random samples (for instance carers attending carers' groups or using respite services), it is difficult to assess just how large an impact differences in sampling will influence the prevalence of psychological ill-health. Notwithstanding this factor, studies of carers in touch with specialist services, such as carers of people attending day hospitals (Gilleard, et al, 1984), or receiving respite services (Levin et al, 1994), have generally reported

higher levels of psychological distress than those found in community samples, such as those derived from GPs' age–sex registers.

While it is clearly important to evaluate services in terms of their effects on carers, there are methodological problems in showing whether or not such services have a beneficial impact. The usefulness of some of the measures used to screen for carer stress has been questioned, in particular for the lack of evidence on their reliability and validity (Vitaliano et al, 1991). The implications of this are important. For instance, a measure with good predictive validity (in other words, the ability to forecast some future event successfully) would be valuable in enabling assistance to be focused on carers at risk while not offering help unnecessarily to carers who feel that they are coping satisfactorily. There are also issues about the cross-cultural validity of some of the instruments.

An alternative, or supplementary, approach is to use a general measure of psychological well being in order to be able to compare carers with similar populations of non-carers (George and Gwyther, 1986). While demonstrable improvements in carers' psychological health would clearly be a desirable outcome of any service intervention, this approach also has its methodological difficulties. Studies have generally reported a wide distribution in initial, or baseline, scores. Some carers report few or no feelings of depression; their scores can only stay the same or worsen. It has been suggested that this effect can lead to the impact of the intervention being underestimated (Whitlach et al, 1991). Equally, other carers are reluctant to accept services until they reach the point at which they have already begun to experience poor psychological health (Moriarty and Levin, 1998). Although day hospital care has been reported to improve psychological health (Gilleard et al, 1984), it is more common to find that those carers who initially have high levels of stress are those who cease caring (Levin et al, 1989, 1994; Wells et al, 1990). These studies have questioned whether quite limited amounts of service receipt would be sufficient to produce reductions in carer stress.

Another study compared carers who received an augmented domiciliary service, in which home support workers provided emotional support, information and advice as well as practical help, with a matched group of carers receiving standard services. It did not find any evidence that the psychological profile of carers in either group had altered. However, receiving the augmented service did mean that people with dementia stayed in the community for longer (Riordan and Bennett, 1998).

Carers who participated in an intensive programme of carer education had significantly lower levels of stress at 12 months than carers of people with dementia who underwent a memory training programme and carers who waited six months before undertaking the carer education programme (Brodaty and Gresham, 1992).

As with entry rates to long-term care, evaluations based solely on whether or not carers continue to care will be incomplete if they do not also consider carers' satisfaction with the help that they receive and take account of the effects of continuing to care when this is not in accordance with carers' wishes.

Views of service users with dementia

Increasingly, we are beginning to accept that attributions of success or failure will be judged differently according to the perspectives of those involved in the evaluation. It is now some years since the absence of views of people receiving care was identified as a limitation within the literature on caring (Barer and Johnson, 1990). While the perspective of service users has been incorporated into most areas of social and healthcare research, these developments remain in their infancy in the field of dementia (Stalker et al, 1999). Of the literature that does exist, more has come from a practice (Goldsmith, 1996) than from a research base. Furthermore, where the approach has been based on interviews with service users, sample sizes have tended to be small. More studies have documented the experiences of people with early dementia (Keady, 1996), but it has also been shown that people with moderate and severe dementia may still have the ability to give their views of services (Bamford, 1998; Levin et al, 1994; Mozley et al, 1999).

Advances in medical research have undoubtedly contributed to improving the public's understanding about dementia and reducing stigma, but it can be argued that the social model of disability is also relevant for dementia care. This approach highlights that it is the attitudes and actions of other people, rather than the features of the disability or disease itself, that disempower people with disabilities. For instance, behaving as if people with dementia are like children (infantilising) has been identified as one of the elements making up the 'malignant social psychology' of dementia care and contributing to a 'loss of personhood' (Kitwood, 1997). The recognition that personhood can be maintained is central to the 'new culture of dementia care' (Kitwood and Bredin, 1992). This approach has been extremely influential in promoting greater recognition for the validity of the views of people with dementia.

Context

At the time that the 1990 NHS and Community Care Act was fully implemented, much uncertainty existed as to how the community care changes would translate into mainstream practice with older people with dementia. First, Challis (1992) had warned that, of the Kent, Gateshead and Darlington case management studies, only the latter provided significant cost savings, and this was because of the high cost of existing long-stay hospital provision. He suggested that the relative price of community and long-term care services within localities could influence the extent to which alternatives to long-term care could be pursued.

Second, in sharp contrast to other groups of people needing care, the general public have tended to see long-term care as a more suitable option for people with dementia (West et al, 1984). As yet, the extent to which changes in approaches to managing risk (Baragwanath, 1997) and improved awareness that people with dementia have service preferences (Goldsmith, 1996) will be reflected in the sort of care that is provided is uncertain.

Third, in identifying the practice skills needed to underpin care management, attention was focused on the negotiation skills necessary in order to work with clients whose cognitive deficits might hinder their ability to participate fully and as equals:

Services to older people with dementia will provide one of the first testing grounds for the new relationship between workers and clients required to carry out effective care management. (Fisher, 1990a, p 240)

At the same time, none of these issues were entirely new. The difficulties in enabling a group at risk of entry to long-term care to live at home, in providing choice to clients who were likely to have difficulties in expressing their preferences, and in balancing the needs and preferences of people with dementia against those of their carers, were all problems that existed before the Act. Their relevance is undiminished as social and healthcare services continue to develop following the White Papers *The new NHS* (Secretary of State for Health, 1997) and *Modernising social services* (Secretary of State for Health, 1998).

Structure of the book

This book provides an account of the key issues and findings from the study. Each chapter deals with a different aspect, but there are themes that overlap between them.

Chapter 2 explains the study design and methods. To avoid repetition in later chapters, readers are encouraged to refer back to this chapter whenever they wish to be reminded of details about the interview schedules and survey instruments. Relevant information is also included the Appendices, and in the Glossary at the beginning of the book.

Chapter 3 reports on sources of referral within the study SSDs, gives case examples to show the different types of referral, describes the characteristics of study participants and summarises what happened to them over the course of the study.

Chapter 4 examines the assessment process and reports on waiting times for assessments, user and carer experiences of assessment, the involvement of other professionals and the provision of care plans.

The role played by carers of people with dementia is crucial, and Chapter 5 highlights their experiences of caring and the contribution they made.

Chapter 6 examines the range of community services that were used and reports on the frequency and length of time for which they were provided each week. Through case examples, it examines how services were combined in care plans and discusses the views of carers and users.

Chapter 7 draws together some of the themes explored in earlier chapters by comparing people who remained at home with those who entered long-term care. Survival analyses are used to explore the interactions between severity of cognitive impairment, access to a carer and the receipt of community services on rates of entry to long-term care. The reactions of the people with dementia towards admission to long-term care are discussed.

Dementia is closely associated with increased use of health and social services and so more stress is being placed on the importance of identifying the costs of different forms of care. There is a need for post-April 1993 data on the costs associated with service use (Kavanagh and Knapp, 1999) and Chapter 8 reports on the costs of participants' packages of care.

Chapter 9, the concluding chapter, draws together the study's findings and highlights some issues that have implications for policy and practice.

The names used in the text are pseudonyms, and no quotations or descriptions of events have been given that might be directly identifiable with any single individual who was interviewed during the course of the study.

Design and methods

Key points

- This chapter highlights some of the practical difficulties in identifying people with dementia referred to SSDs and describes the measures used in the study.

- The sampling frame was drawn from the records of 14 social work teams across three different SSDs and involved identifying people with dementia aged 65 and over who had been assessed.

- Separate interviews took place with assessors (*n*=206), proxy informants, such as staff working in residential homes (*n*=34), carers (*n*=103) and people with dementia (*n*=122).

- Proxy informants (*n*=38), carers (*n*=89), and people with dementia (*n*=93) were re-interviewed an average of 11 months later.

"[I'd] like some sort of advice [about the] best way of planning for the future though that's out of my hands. I don't know. [I'm] very worried and a bit resentful that I can't find help." (Mrs Jacob, interviewed at Time One)

"I think a year on, your ideas harden and clarify.... What we owe them [people with dementia] is quality of life, not just existence ... know that since I talked to you last, a lot's in place but it's just she's [mother's] your life. It governs everything. I do now sometimes wonder what

would have happened if I hadn't been here. Would more [community] care have been given or would she have been taken into care?" (Mrs Jacob, interviewed at Time Two)

Introduction

There are methodological and practical difficulties in identifying people with dementia in SSD populations.

While it is possible to estimate the likely prevalence of people with dementia within the geographical area covered by each SSD, there has been very little research into the prevalence of psychiatric disorder among actual SSD clients aged over 65 (Banerjee, 1993). The available literature demonstrates that long-term care settings are comparatively well researched compared with people using community services, such as home care.

It would be feasible to screen every client or resident for evidence of cognitive impairment in studies based on samples drawn from a single social work team or from residents of a particular home. However, few studies have attempted to identify people with dementia across whole SSD populations. The reasons for this appear to be largely logistical. The majority of SSD adult clients are over the age of 65. Over a six-month period in 1996, the average rate of referrals in a sample of 39 SSDs was 164 per 1,000 of the population aged 65 and over (Edwards and Kenny, 1997).

Two studies have identified people with dementia using a service-based census in which workers were asked to identify clients on their caseload whom they believed to have features suggestive of dementia (Levin et al, 1989; Carr, 1992). While clearly not adequate for epidemiological and clinical research, the low cost and the relative speed with which a census can be completed make them a pragmatic solution in some circumstances (Gordon et al, 1997).

Another method has been to use the case review forms originally designed by Goldberg and Warburton (1979), or variants on them. These forms are designed to be completed by fieldworkers for all clients with whom they are currently involved. They describe the client's problems, the type of help provided, the changes achieved and plans for the future.

However, the approaches outlined above share the weaknesses of sampling strategies that involve asking workers to provide details of clients who meet certain criteria.

First, the degree of cooperation from individual practitioners will vary. For instance, Petch and colleagues (1996) used a variant on the case review system. They reported that nine out of 65 practitioners in their study failed to make any returns, and the final sample size would appear to indicate that not everyone met the original target of providing a case review form for each of their last five or six assessments.

Second, researchers have no means of identifying whether everyone for whom a return should have been made has been included, although sampling from multiple service points may result in people excluded by one organisation or in an individual being picked up in returns from another (Spicker and Gordon, 1997).

Third, the accuracy of asking health, social services and voluntary organisations to pre-select people with dementia from among all those with whom they are in contact is conditional upon their ability to identify every client for whom they should provide details. While we have some evidence on the recognition of dementia in primary care settings (O'Connor et al, 1988; Iliffe et al, 1994), there is

almost none on social workers' ability to recognise possible dementia or the frequency with which they routinely screen for cognitive impairment.

O'Connor and colleagues (1989b) and Carr (1992) have both suggested that social workers tend to view dementia more in terms of its severe manifestations. By implication, it is possible that some social workers may not recognise signs of mild or moderate dementia in their clients. Using the Survey Psychiatric Assessment Schedule (SPAS) (Bond et al, 1980), Cohen and Fisher (1987) identified probable dementia in 44% (n=49) of 112 SSD clients aged 70 and over. Of these, 32 had been identified by social workers as having dementia, giving a 'correct identification' rate of 65%.

How do these recognition rates compare with those made by other professionals? O'Connor and colleagues (1988) found recognition rates of 58% among GPs and 84% among community nurses. Harwood and colleagues (1997) suggested that 84% of patients with cognitive impairment on medical wards were identified as such by physicians. However, each of these studies used different ways of screening for dementia, so we should be very cautious in drawing comparisons between them.

The Social Services Inspectorate (SSI) (1997) has pointed to the difficulties in using SSD information systems as a means of extracting data about the numbers of people with dementia who were using services. Many SSDs did not introduce fully computerised information systems until the implementation of the 1990 NHS and Community Care Act. How they define and record referrals or assessments and make links between written case records and computerised information varies across departments (Barnes, 1996; Spackman et al, 1997). Depending on the information system in use, there are different ways of categorising clients. Thus, categories such as 'older people', 'frail elderly', 'mental health' and 'elderly mentally ill' (EMI) might all include individuals with dementia.

An issue that appears to be reported more frequently in research carried out in SSDs and voluntary organisations than in health settings is that of workers requesting that certain clients be excluded from the study (Hatfield et al, 1994; Cumella et al, 1996; Leek and Fletcher, 1996).

Practitioners may consider that there are circumstances in which participation in a study in which there are no direct benefits may not be advisable for their clients (Challis and Darton, 1990).

Some studies of community-based samples of people with dementia have recorded use of SSD services (O'Connor et al, 1989b; Livingston et al, 1990, 1997). This reduces the likelihood of sample selection bias, but the resulting relatively low yield of service users limits the type of statistical analyses that can be completed (Banerjee and Macdonald, 1996). The focus of these studies is such that they tend to record what was received without reporting on the types and intensity of service packages or providing detailed consumer perspectives.

The community care changes highlighted the need for more information on how SSDs were approaching the care of people with dementia. The stress laid on assessment suggested that this was a crucial area on which to focus. However, existing research indicated that, if we intended to concentrate on people with dementia who had received an SSD assessment, there would be no established satisfactory design from which to recruit a sample of a size with sufficient analytic power.

Summary of design and methods

The study was based on a sample of people who were referred to 14 social work teams within three SSDs between 1 November 1994 and 28 February 1995 and who went on to receive an assessment. Figure 2.1 (p 14) summarises how the sample was selected and outlines each stage of the study.

Information was collected through a series of separate interviews with assessors, carers, proxy informants and people with dementia. Carers, proxy informants and people with dementia were re-interviewed, on average, 11 months later. The timespan during which data collection took place is shown in Table 2.1.

SSDs and types of social work team included

Three SSDs agreed to take part in the research. Approval was sought from the ADSS Service Evaluation, Research and Information Committee and from the appropriate local research ethics committees. Elsewhere, we have explained that the study SSDs were *alike* in that the percentage of the population in the 65-and-over age group and the proportion of older people living alone were similar. They *differed* in that each was an example of the type of local authority that existed at the time (county council, metropolitan borough, inner London borough), in the areas that they covered (urban and rural) and in the way that social work teams were organised (area, hospital, and specialist teams for older people with mental health problems) (Moriarty and Webb, 1995).

At the time, a total of 22 social work teams covered the geographical areas included in the study. They consisted of 13 area teams dealing with all older people, seven specialist teams for older people with mental health problems, and two teams based in acute hospitals. In the metropolitan borough, older people were seen by one of three area teams and a hospital social work team.

Table 2.1: Data collection

Period of collection	Information collected
November 1994-March 1995	Information on referrals made to the participating teams
March 1995-August 1995	Interview assessor to establish the person's eligibility for the study and to find out more detailed information on the referral, assessment and circumstances of the older person
April 1995-December 1995	First set of interviews (Time One) with the older person, his or her carer or a suitable proxy informant
November 1995-December 1996	Second set of interviews (Time Two) with the older person, his or her carer or a suitable proxy informant

Figure 2.1: Outline of the study stages

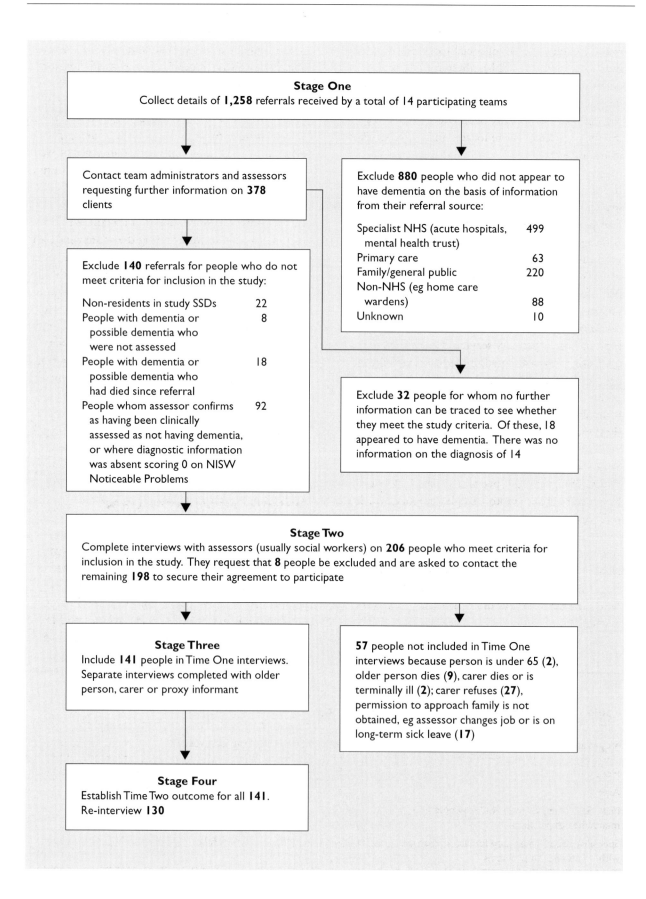

Stage One
Collect details of **1,258** referrals received by a total of 14 participating teams

Contact team administrators and assessors requesting further information on **378** clients

Exclude **880** people who did not appear to have dementia on the basis of information from their referral source:

Specialist NHS (acute hospitals, mental health trust)	499
Primary care	63
Family/general public	220
Non-NHS (eg home care wardens)	88
Unknown	10

Exclude **140** referrals for people who do not meet criteria for inclusion in the study:

Non-residents in study SSDs	22
People with dementia or possible dementia who were not assessed	8
People with dementia or possible dementia who had died since referral	18
People whom assessor confirms as having been clinically assessed as not having dementia, or where diagnostic information was absent scoring 0 on NISW Noticeable Problems	92

Exclude **32** people for whom no further information can be traced to see whether they meet the study criteria. Of these, 18 appeared to have dementia. There was no information on the diagnosis of 14

Stage Two
Complete interviews with assessors (usually social workers) on **206** people who meet criteria for inclusion in the study. They request that **8** people be excluded and are asked to contact the remaining **198** to secure their agreement to participate

Stage Three
Include **141** people in Time One interviews. Separate interviews completed with older person, carer or proxy informant

57 people not included in Time One interviews because person is under 65 (**2**), older person dies (**9**), carer dies or is terminally ill (**2**); carer refuses (**27**), permission to approach family is not obtained, eg assessor changes job or is on long-term sick leave (**17**)

Stage Four
Establish Time Two outcome for all **141**.
Re-interview **130**

This was also the model that prevailed in the northern part of the county council. In one district in the southern half of the county, a pioneering multidisciplinary team of social workers, community psychiatric nurses (CPNs), physiotherapists and occupational therapists (OTs) had been set up to deal with older people with mental health problems. This model had recently been extended. Some of the specialist teams were located in hospitals, others in resource centres.

In the London borough, a system of primary and specialist social work teams operated. There were four primary teams and two specialist teams. Although the primary teams did deal with clients with mental health problems, they referred the more severe or complex cases to the appropriate specialist team for their catchment area. In contrast to the county council, these teams were made up of social workers, but both teams worked closely with the local old age psychiatry service. One of the specialist teams was based in the local mental health trust and the other was situated adjacent to the area office, although some of the social workers in this team also had offices in the mental health trust for their locality.

Unless the text indicates the contrary, the multidisciplinary and specialist social work teams have been collapsed into a single category, which we refer to as 'specialist'.

Arrangements in the study SSDs have since been altered to some degree as a result of reorganisation, an issue that was also identified in a study of social work practitioners and their managers (Levin and Webb, 1997).

In order to avoid the potential sample selection bias of including only those people pre-identified by the social workers as having suspected dementia, we wanted information on everybody over the age of 65 who had been assessed. However, the London and metropolitan boroughs and the part of the county council included in the study each served populations of over 200,000 people, of whom about 15% were aged 65 and over. The volume of likely referrals over a four-month period meant that we did not have the resources to collect records from all 22 teams.

As the other two study areas were urban, we included all the teams covering the more rural parts of the county but excluded area teams where specialist multidisciplinary teams existed. In the London borough, we included the specialist teams only. All teams in the metropolitan borough were included. The teams varied in size from two hospital social work teams based in large district general hospitals to specialist multidisciplinary teams covering rural districts in which there was only a single social worker.

Table 2.2 lists the types of team that were represented in the study.

Sample recruitment and selection

The team managers warned us that asking social workers and other staff to complete additional lengthy forms would reduce the degree of cooperation that we could expect. Therefore, we used pre-existing record-keeping systems within each team and collected details of clients aged 65

Table 2.2: Types of team participating in the study

Type of team	n	Study area
Hospital	2	Metropolitan borough (1) and county (1)
Area	4	Metropolitan borough (3) and county (1)
Multidisciplinary team for older people with mental health problems	6	County
Specialist social work team for older people with mental health problems	2	London borough

and over referred over a four-month period from a combination of sources: the local authority computerised information system; records of allocation meetings; referral forms; referral books and lists. All four area teams, both hospital teams, and four of the eight specialist teams, gave us either a copy of the original referral, access to the referral book, or a list of referrals downloaded from the information system. The remaining four specialist teams provided details of people aged 65 and over who had gone on to receive an assessment.

From Figure 2.1, it can be seen that we collected details of 1,258 people who were referred to the 14 teams participating in the study over a four-month period. This represented a total of 1,342 referrals, as 67 people were referred twice, seven people were referred three times, and one person was referred four times.

We screened the referral information for evidence of diagnoses of a form of dementia, unspecified mental health problems, references to cognitive impairment, short-term memory loss, confusion and instances of self-neglect or unsafe or unusual behaviour. Once we identified referrals of this kind, we contacted the social worker to whom they had been allocated. The number of people on whom we requested further information was 378.

The purpose of this stage was to clarify whether or not the person referred met the criteria for inclusion in the study. These were that he or she was:

- aged 65 or over at the time of referral;
- had signs of cognitive impairment that were suggestive of dementia;
- had gone on to receive an assessment after referral to social services.

Anybody who had died since referral or who lived outside the study SSDs was automatically excluded. If the social worker could confirm that someone had been clinically assessed (that is, by an old age psychiatrist, other specialist or their GP) as *not* having dementia, then that person was also excluded. If the social worker did not know whether or not the person referred had been clinically assessed, then we completed the NISW Noticeable Problems (Levin et al, 1989). This is a

six-item informant questionnaire designed to establish whether the subject of the questions has any cognitive impairment. Scores on these questions can be treated either as a continuous variable (1-6) or as a categorical variable: mild (1-2), moderate (3-4) and severe (5-6). They have been shown to correlate well with diagnoses made by old age psychiatrists using the Copeland et al (1976) Geriatric Mental State Schedule (GMS) (see Graham and Waldron, 1983). The full set of questions is included in Appendix 2. People scoring 0 on the NISW Noticeable Problems (*n*=28) were also excluded.

In the context that not every referral to an SSD necessarily results in an assessment, concern has been expressed about the way in which assessments may be linked to budget considerations and limited to those identified as being 'at risk' (Davis et al, 1998). Among the 378 people about whom we made enquiries, we identified 15 people, of whom eight appeared to have dementia or possible dementia, who did not go on to receive an assessment. Of the eight, two were passed on to another professional, and three carers and two older people refused to be assessed. While it appeared that this group represented a small proportion of referrals to the teams from which we did have information, as there were four teams from whom we did not have details of every referral, this figure potentially underestimates the number of people with dementia who were referred but not assessed.

There were 32 clients for whom we could not trace further information and so were unable to determine whether or not they should have been included in the study.

SSD policies on client confidentiality meant that we could not access potential study participants without their prior permission. Once we had established that someone was eligible for the study, we requested that the assessor approach the family for their permission to contact them. Suitable proxy informants, such as staff in residential or nursing homes or wardens, were identified for people without carers. Four people had no identified carer or proxy informant. In their case, we were given permission to approach them directly and all agreed to participate. All study participants were sent a letter inviting them to participate which told them the name of the interviewer who would be contacting them and included an information leaflet about the study.

The number of people from whom we collected data and the number of people for whom insufficient information was available to determine whether or not they met criteria for inclusion in the study could have been reduced by including only active or open cases, that is people who were currently receiving input from an assessor. However, Brown and colleagues (1996) have shown that there is a difference between current caseload clients and the overall referral population. We balanced the disadvantages of losing potential study participants through staff changes or the non-tracing of records against the advantages of including a wider range of clients, including people who refused services or self-funding residents in long-term care.

We had originally intended to screen a number of referrals to area and hospital teams who were *not* identified as having dementia for evidence of cognitive impairment. This was to check whether our sampling methods meant that we were mistakenly excluding people from the study. (The nature of the way that the specialist teams operated was such that it was highly unlikely that we omitted any of the people with dementia whom they had seen.) There is no doubt that such an approach would have added to the study's rigour. In the event, the work involved in setting up and maintaining the sample meant that it would have been impossible to achieve both elements if we were to complete the study within the funding period.

Response rate

We decided to include five of the nine people selected for pilot interview in the main study after we had checked that they did not differ in any way from the other participants. Table 2.3 shows the survey response rate both inclusive and exclusive of the 32 people for whom we could not obtain the full information to determine whether they were eligible cases. The *lower* range assumes that all 32 untraced people should have been included in the study. The *upper* range assumes that none of the 32

would have been eligible. The actual study response rate is likely to lie somewhere between the two. Assuming that all 32 untraced people would have been eligible for the study, the Time One response rate of 62% is slightly lower than similar studies (Qureshi and Walker, 1989; Buck et al, 1997; Philp et al, 1997).

The study response rate should not be confused with the respondent response rate, that is, the response rate among people who were actually approached for an interview. The response rate of 84% among the people who were actually approached for an interview (see Figure 2.1) is very similar to those reported in other studies. It should be considered in the context that many of the older people and their carers had just undergone potentially stressful events, such as moves to long-term care, and the study did not offer any direct benefit to participants in the form of access to diagnostic services, medical treatment or other help. Furthermore, as we show later, the interview schedule was complex and time consuming. Therefore, we felt that it would be unethical to use techniques aimed at increasing the response rate, such as re-contacting people who had already refused or allocating them to a different interviewer.

Data from the assessors' interviews were used to compare the 141 people who took part in the Time One interviews with the remaining 65 who did not (see Figure 2.1). On the basis of age, gender, degree of cognitive impairment as measured by the NISW noticeable problems and whether or not they had a carer, the characteristics of the 141 participants did not appear to differ from the 65 non-participants (see Appendix 1). However, the small numbers in the comparison group mean that there is a possibility of Type II errors. (Tests carried out on small samples sometimes lead to the null hypothesis that there is no difference between two groups being accepted when, in reality, it is false and the groups *are* different.)

Table 2.3: Survey response rate*

Study stage	Range	*n* eligible	*n* interview	*% response*
Assessor interview	Lower	238	206	87
	Upper	206	206	100
Time One interview	Lower	227	141	62
	Upper	195	141	72
Time Two interview	Lower	141	130	92
	Upper	141	130	92

* See text for explanation of upper and lower ranges.

Interviews with assessors

Full details of this stage of the study have been discussed elsewhere (Moriarty and Webb, 1995). Excluding enquiries about their clients who did not meet the study criteria (covered in the section on sample recruitment and selection), a total of 206 interviews were completed with 65 different assessors, either face-to-face or over the telephone. Each assessor was asked about a mean number of three clients (standard deviation [SD] 2). Assessors were interviewed approximately four-and-a-half months after the referral (SD 60 days) and three-and-a-half months after the assessment (SD 67 days). Appointments for face-to-face or telephone interviews with assessors were made in advance to enable them to access records or check any relevant details beforehand. Almost all the assessors were qualified social workers, but some staff without a social work qualification, such as community care assistants or home care organisers, were also interviewed.

As we discussed in the section on sample recruitment and selection, assessors were asked if they knew whether the older person's mental state had been clinically assessed, and they completed the NISW Noticeable Problems (Levin et al, 1989). We also collected information on the circumstances surrounding the referral, support from carers and other family members, the assessment itself, and what services were being provided.

Time One interviews with carers and proxy informants

One hundred and two carers and 34 proxy informants were interviewed for the first time, on average, six-and-a-quarter months after the referral (SD 76 days) and five-and-a-quarter months after the assessment (SD 78 days).

Overall, three quarters of the older people had been identified as having a carer. This was defined as someone who, at the time of referral, was giving unpaid assistance with one or more activities of daily living (ADLs) or instrumental activities of daily living (IADLs) at least once a week. There are different ways of defining ADLs and IADLs, but in this study ADLs were defined as transfer, washing, bathing, dressing, using the lavatory, eating, getting up and going to bed, self-medicating and leaving the house (10 items) and IADLs as shopping, housework, food preparation, laundry, household maintenance and managing money (six items) (Levin et al, 1989).

A third of the carers were co-resident (*n*=30); that is, they lived in the same household as the person for whom they cared; 40% were non-resident (*n*=41). They made an average of eight visits per week (SD 9) to the older people. The remainder (*n*=32) were former carers. This is an unsatisfactory term but we used it to distinguish between carers of people living in long-term care at Time One and those caring for someone living in the community. The mean number of visits made by former carers to the older person per week was three (SD 3) and, as Chapter 5 explains, many continued to be closely involved in day-to-day care. At 31% (*n*=10), the proportion of former carers who had lived with the older person was slightly lower than the proportion of co-resident carers among those who were currently caring.

Although we interviewed a total of 102 carers, the number of older people with carers was 103 because one man living in the community and one woman resident in long-term care were cared for by their daughter who acted as a double informant.

Proxy informants were defined as people giving paid care to the older person or giving unpaid assistance but not at the level of a carer. The literature shows that it is rare for anyone other than kin to be involved in giving unpaid personal care (Arber and Ginn, 1991; Wenger, 1992; Parker and Lawton, 1994). Excluding paid staff, only three of the proxy informants and two of the carers were not related to the person for whom they cared; 23 proxy informants were staff working full-time in long-term care settings who reported that they saw the older person almost every day.

The carers and proxy informants were interviewed in order to find out details of the help that the person with dementia received in completing the ADLs and IADLs described above. The Lambeth Disability Questionnaire (Charlton et al, 1983) was also administered. The presence of non-cognitive features of dementia was recorded by asking questions on behavioural problems, aggression and personality traits devised by Enid Levin (Levin et al, 1989). Both carers and proxy informants answered detailed questions about the assessment and the services received. They were also asked about their role and experiences of caring for the person with dementia.

Specific sections for carers recorded information on their demographic details, self-reported health, opportunities for leisure, recent life events and social support. They also completed the 28-item GHQ (GHQ-28) (Goldberg and Williams, 1988), a well validated screening instrument for anxiety and depression which has been widely used in studies of this sort. In common with all screening questionnaires, the GHQ does not make clinical diagnoses, but people with scores in excess of the cut-point (we used 6+) are likely to be experiencing symptoms associated with psychiatric illnesses, such as depression and anxiety.

We asked about the older person's last main occupation and the carer's current or last occupation using the 'conventional approach' (Arber and Ginn, 1992) based on the last known occupation of the head of the household. Socio-economic groups (SEGs) were classified into five social classes. Household and, where possible, individual social class were assigned (OPCS, 1990).

On average, interviews with a proxy informant lasted 45 minutes. Those with carers took an average of one hour and 40 minutes. Interviews with current carers took about 20 minutes longer than those with former carers because additional sections on the use of community services were completed.

Time One interviews with the older people

One hundred and twenty-two older people were interviewed separately in order to screen for dementia and depression and to find out their views of services. The remaining 19 older people in the study were not interviewed, mainly because their carers were concerned that they might become upset by being asked questions designed to assess their level of cognitive impairment.

Interviewing people with dementia raises additional ethical dilemmas. The Helsinki declaration states that in medical research:

Each potential subject must be adequately informed of the aims, methods, anticipated benefits and potential hazards of the study, and the discomfort it may entail. He or she should be informed that he or she is at liberty to abstain from participation in the study, and that he or she is free to withdraw his or her consent to participation at any time. The physician should then obtain the subject's freely-given informed consent, preferably in writing. (Declaration of Helsinki, 1964)

It does, however, also allow for circumstances in which informed consent does not need to be sought and for circumstances where participants are judged to be incompetent and consent can be sought from the person's legal guardian. It is clear that a person's ability to give informed consent in the fullest sense will be affected by dementia. At the same time, some decision-making capacity may be retained (Schaum Resau, 1995). In circumstances such as these, there is clearly no simple answer. Much depends on the type of study that is being undertaken. Generally, lower levels of consent have been deemed to be acceptable when the research does not involve any additional procedures than when it is part of a clinical trial (Goodacre and Smith, 1997).

There is now a well argued case for involving service users in research, not only on ethical grounds, but also because of the technical benefits (Fisher, 1998). Excluding older people with dementia from the process of reporting their experiences directly themselves has meant that family and paid carers have often been the only source of information on their views. Our previous experience had suggested that the ability of older people with moderate and severe dementia to give their opinions themselves may be underestimated. In a study of people with dementia using respite services, we found that many of them had very definite views about the gains and disadvantages of using the different services. In some cases their views coincided with those of their carers; in others they differed (Levin et al, 1994). We decided that the arguments in favour of including the direct views of people with dementia outweighed those based on concerns that not everyone interviewed would understand the nature and purpose of the research.

In addition to the question of consent, another consideration stemmed from our knowledge that being asked questions designed to test the level of cognitive ability can sometimes cause embarrassment and anxiety (Tinker, 1997). One solution is to omit such questions altogether from the interview process. However, this removes any means of being able to analyse participants' comments in relation to their severity of cognitive impairment. It also indirectly helps to perpetuate the notion that people with dementia cannot give their views because it can offer no evidence on the severity of cognitive impairment that has to be present before a person is no longer interviewable.

Forty per cent (*n*=48) of the older people interviewed gave their written consent. The remainder were no longer able to write and verbally agreed to take part. In these circumstances, their carer or proxy informant was asked to sign a form confirming that the older person had been given a full explanation of the purpose of the study and what was involved. The interviewers were instructed to stop interviewing whenever an older person who had initially consented to take part started to demonstrate their unwillingness to continue, either verbally or non-verbally. Four interviews were ended this way.

Although interviews with the older people were completed separately from those with carers and proxy informants, only 45% of the older people were interviewed on their own with no one else present. As with any research that takes place in private households, researchers have very limited means of influencing whether any one else is in the room when participants are being interviewed. One solution would have been for two interviewers to visit and to interview the carer or proxy and the older person in separate rooms, but this would have doubled the interviewing costs.

We asked the interviewers to record in their notes whether factors such as the presence of another person, the timing or location of the interview had influenced the interview with the older person. In four instances they reported that the older person had appealed to the carer for help with answers to questions. In another four cases the carer or proxy had well-meaningly tried to prompt the older person. These eight cases represent a very small proportion of the 122 older people interviews. It suggests that, while there is no way of knowing whether or not the presence of another person influenced the content of the older person's replies, the vast majority of carers and proxy informants seemed to be aware of the purpose of having separate interviews and did not try to intervene when the older person was being interviewed.

After reviewing various instruments to screen for cognitive impairment (Moriarty et al, 1994), we selected the Brief Assessment Schedule (BAS) (Macdonald et al, 1982), which comprises items from the Comprehensive Assessment and Referral Evaluation (CARE) interview schedule (Golden et al, 1984) and tests for the presence and severity of dementia using the Organic Brain Scale (OBS) and for the presence of depression using the Depression Scale (DEP). Scores on the OBS range from 0-8. A cut-point of 2 or 3 was found useful as a screen for dementia in a survey of community and long-term care residents (Macdonald et al, 1982). A maximum score of 8 has been shown to predict a diagnosis of severe dementia in a sample of people in long-term care with a sensitivity of 94% and a specificity of 69% (Mann et al, 1984). Scores on the DEP range from 0 to 24. A cut-point of 6 or 7 out of a maximum score of 24 has been demonstrated to accord with a psychiatrist's diagnosis of depression made independently using DSM III R criteria with a sensitivity of 89% and a specificity of 81% (Allen et al, 1994). The BAS schedule has an introductory filter section, designed to deal with respondents who have very severe levels of impairment. If an informant is unable to answer any of four filter questions correctly, the schedule is terminated. This means that the DEP questions are omitted and the respondent is given a maximum score of 8 on the OBS. Good rates of inter-rater reliability with the BAS have been reported (Gurland et al, 1979; Mann et al, 1989).

The final part of the interview involved asking the older people about their experiences of assessment and services and briefly discussing their past history and family. This section was completed with all participants who were interviewed, even those who had not been able to answer the BAS filter questions correctly. The average length of a complete interview with a person with dementia lasted about half an hour. A summary of the three different schedules used with carers, proxy informants and older people is included in Appendix 3.

Time Two interviews

Second interviews with the carers, proxy informants and older people were completed just under 11 months later (SD 103 days) and the main measures repeated. Ninety per cent of these interviews were carried out by the interviewer who had completed the Time One interview. Information on service use was collected again in order to identify services that (a) had been used continuously between Times One and Two; (b) had started since Time One; (c)

had stopped by Time Two; or (d) had not been used throughout the study. On average, proxy interviews lasted around 35 minutes and carer interviews around an hour and a quarter. Full interviews with the older people lasted about 25 minutes. As was to be expected, the proportion of older person interviews in which the BAS was terminated after the filter questions increased from around 30% to 40%. We were able to establish data for key variables – continued residence in the community, date of admission to long-term care or death – for all 141 participants. The re-interview rate for the 141 cases included in the study was high (92%).

Interviewer training

We completed almost 10% of Time One and Time Two interviews with carers, proxies and older people ourselves. However, the majority were carried out by a team of interviewers whom we had recruited and trained. All had backgrounds that gave them considerable experience in interviewing older people and/or carers in a research or other professional capacity. The interviewers were also issued with a set of detailed guidelines covering ethical issues, potential difficulties while interviewing, advice on interviewing people with dementia, and instructions for completing and coding specific items.

The completion of detailed and complicated interview schedules, in addition to the low numbers of people who refused to participate when contacted by the interviewers and the high re-interview rates, are indications of the interviewers' skill and hard work.

Discussion on methods of sample selection

The study involved following up a group of people with dementia over an average of 18 months. Assessors, carers, proxy informants and older people with dementia were interviewed separately. The re-interview rate was high. However, there are issues in sample recruitment and selection that need to be addressed.

There is comparatively less information on the use of social care services by people with dementia than on their use of health services. In view of this, and taking account of the new responsibilities given to SSDs by the 1990 NHS and Community Care Act, the study was designed to concentrate on people who had received an SSD assessment. We identified a small group of people with dementia or possible dementia (*n*=8) who were referred but not assessed, but they were not included in subsequent stages.

There are difficulties in identifying people with dementia within SSD populations when the design does not involve screening every potential study participant. The methods of sample selection meant that it was possible that some people assigned to the non-dementia group should have been included in the study.

Within the study areas, there will, of course, have been a group of people with dementia who had been assessed by primary or secondary healthcare services but who were not referred on to their SSD. Interviewing staff across agencies and tracking service contacts can be a lengthy and complex process (Petch et al, 1996). Table 2.1 shows how much of the data collection period was allocated to sample recruitment. We were concerned that any actions that might have extended this stage of the study would compromise our ability to achieve two sets of interviews with older people, carers and proxy informants within the funding period.

The study does not claim to be generalisable. Only three SSDs were involved and there was only one department in which all the social work teams were included. The lack of information on the prevalence of people with dementia in all SSDs gives us no means of knowing whether the proportion of people seen by the teams included in the study reflects that to be found in other SSDs serving similar populations.

At the same time, it is important to recognise that managers, assessors, clerical and administrative staff set aside considerable time in order for the project to go ahead, and we had to find ways of sample selection that would not cause still further demands on their workload and even run the risk that they would decide to withdraw from the study. The approach we adopted would seem to have been expedient, given other accounts reporting social workers' concerns about increased paperwork and bureaucracy which they attribute to the community care changes (Lewis and Glennerster, 1996; Petch et al, 1996; Levin and Webb, 1997). As we hope will be evident from later chapters, the design enabled us to examine assessment and the provision of services from different perspectives (carers, people with dementia and service providers in the form of many of the proxy informants). It included people who were living at home and in long-term care and supported the use of a range of statistical analyses. The follow-up enabled us to look at changes over time. This is discussed in the next chapter, in which we report on what happened to the older people over the course of the study.

The older people in the study

Key points

- **This chapter describes the circumstances under which the 141 older people included in the study had been referred to the SSD and summarises what happened to them over the following year and a half.**

- **Many people had been referred by their carer or another family member.**

- **Few referrals identified short-term issues; the majority indicated a need for long-term support.**

- **The overall trend was towards admission to long-term care, but there was volatility between community, hospital, and long-term care settings, particularly in the first few months after referral.**

- **Case studies are used to show some of the different pathways between community and long-term care that were taken as a result of referral to the SSD.**

"I'm a very happy creature. [I've got] nothing to be sad about. I've got my home and I don't want for anything. I live alone, but it doesn't worry me. Life is what you make it." (Miss Bertram, living alone in the London borough)

This chapter sets out the framework for the remainder of the book by describing the older people included in the study and showing what happened to them over the course of the following year and a half. Before doing this, we must first consider the circumstances that had led to their referral to the SSD.

Referral sources and reasons for referral

The single largest source of referral was the NHS. Thirty-two per cent of study participants had been referred by secondary healthcare providers; in most cases, these referrals had been made while they were hospital inpatients. Of the rest, 14% had been referred by primary care, 30% had been made by family members or the general public and the remaining 24% resulted from referrals from other social care agencies such as home care, day care and wardens.

Information on the circumstances that had precipitated the referral was used to develop a typology of referral categories. Not all referrals were easy to categorise; sometimes they had occurred after a combination of events or for several reasons.

Case example

Mrs Raymond had been assessed by an old age psychiatrist, who concluded that she was in the early stages of dementia. Shortly afterwards, she was admitted to hospital with chest pain and investigations showed that she had suffered a heart attack. She was referred to the social worker in order to see what help she and her husband would require on discharge.

In this case, the referral reflected the way in which people with dementia may have multiple difficulties, including needs for both health and social care.

It was not always possible to make each category mutually exclusive.

Case example

Mrs Quentin had expressed paranoid ideas and behaved aggressively towards her husband. When she threatened to leave the house, the emergency GP was called out and she was referred to the SSD. The assessor explained that, while the referral had originated from concern about the immediate safety of Mrs Quentin, in reality it reflected the underlying long-term problem that Mr Quentin had been looking after his wife, who had severe dementia, for several years without any support other than from his son who lived some distance away.

In occurrences such as this, categories were assigned on the basis of what appeared to be the *primary* reason for the referral.

About a fifth of the referrals were concerned with the immediate needs of the older person, including fears for their safety and concerns about self-neglect. It was clear that many of the referrals made for people living alone fell into this category.

Case example

Mrs Benedict's daughter described how she reached the decision to refer her mother to the SSD when her mother came to stay with the family. "At Christmas I realised she was not doing what I thought she was. [She was] always very good at covering up. The Thursday before Christmas she had fallen and was very bruised. She looked as if she'd been mugged. After Christmas, I rang social services and asked for a care package."

Another fifth of the referrals suggested a need for more support. Here, the intention was to maintain the status quo by using services in a preventative way.

Case example

Although she lived some distance away, Mrs Cecil had been caring for her father for three years "because he needed it. [He has] severe forgetfulness." It had been her own idea to initiate the referral. "[I] rang up [social services] to find things out. About home help."

About a third of referrals identified issues associated with caring. Sometimes this was because the carer needed help temporarily while in hospital or during a holiday. Others indicated a need for more long-term support.

Case example

Mrs Walter had been caring for her husband at home with no services. Their only daughter lived locally. While she saw her parents regularly, her own family responsibilities and circumstances limited the support that she could give. Mrs Walter described caring as 'a struggle'. Her feelings were acknowledged by her GP, who referred the couple to the SSD. "The doctor said, 'It's not your husband that needs looking after, it's you. You're the carer'."

This category included a number of cases where the carer did not feel able to continue being the person responsible for full-time care or was prevented from doing so by illness.

Case example

Mrs Miles had been visiting her mother-in-law four times a day for the previous two years. Following an incident at home, Mrs Miles telephoned the GP. The social worker said that she was "at her wits' end" and Mrs Miles described herself as "frantic".

About a tenth of study participants had been referred to the SSD with a request to arrange hospital discharge.

The remainder were a miscellaneous selection of requests for help with finance, accommodation, transfers between social work teams and issues about service provision.

It was also possible to differentiate between referrals that had occurred at times of crisis and those that had not. Where referrals had occurred to give more support to the older person or the carer, only a handful subsequently resulted in an admission to long-term care. By contrast, where they centred on concerns about safety or sudden breakdowns in caring support, well over a half subsequently resulted in admissions to long-term care within a few months. This highlights the way in which the referral circumstances of the older people were intrinsically caught up in issues such as the referring agency's interpretation of the acceptable level of risk. It also demonstrates the need to ensure that the service is balanced so that it can be reactive to short-term risk but proactive in regard to long-term prevention.

The location of the older people during the study

Figure 3.1 shows the location of the 141 participants at referral, assessment and the Time One and Time Two interviews. Two findings are immediately apparent: first, the considerable changes that many study participants experienced over a relatively short time and, second, that the overall trend was towards long-term residential or nursing care.

Figure 3.1: The location of the older people at referral, assessment, Time One and Time Two

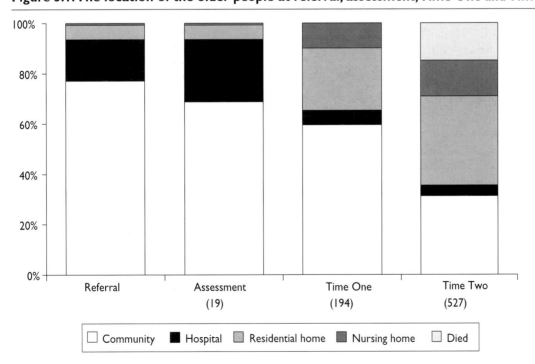

Note: The figures in brackets refer to the average number of days between each time point.

About three quarters of referrals were made for people who were living in the community (*n*=109). A small group (*n*=9) was already living in long-term care and did not return to the community during the course of the study. Around a sixth (*n*=23) were referred when they were in hospital.

By the time of the assessment, on average three weeks later, the number in hospital had risen to 35. This was because 11 people living at home and one person living in residential care at the time of their referral were subsequently admitted to hospital.

Events occurring between referral and admission suggested that these admissions were not avoidable, in the sense that delays between referral and assessment had led to a deterioration in the situation. For instance, one woman was admitted to hospital with chest pain and shortness of breath. In other cases, the carer had a sudden illness. However, in circumstances where carers become ill or the person with dementia develops a sudden temporary increased need for care, some parts of the country are able to offer a domiciliary crisis care service. These have been presented as a more suitable solution than institutional emergency care and may reduce the high rates of long-term care that occur with this group (Bartlett, 1996).

As Chapters 6 and 8 both show, study participants received very limited levels of home care, home-based carer support and community nursing services. Providing the intensity of service that would enable older people with dementia to remain at home in these sorts of circumstances would require considerable investment on the part of both health and social services. It may explain why home-based crisis or emergency provision continues to be outside the mainstream.

When the Time One interviews with the older people and carers or proxy informants took place, approximately five months after the assessment, the number of people still living in the community was 84. The group consisted of 71 people who had been assessed at home and 13 who had returned home following hospital discharge; 21 people in hospital when they were assessed had moved to long-term care; 27 people had been referred and assessed at home but had moved into long-term care.

Approximately 11 months on, when the Time Two interviews took place, almost 15% of the sample (*n*=21) had died. This was a lower proportion than in a study with a broadly similar design but with a higher proportion of people with severe dementia (Levin et al, 1994). Less than a third of the original 141 participants were still at home (*n*=44). Chapter 7 discusses in more detail why some people remained at home while others entered long-term care.

Demographic characteristics of the older people

In order to understand the factors determining whether or not people stayed at home, it is important to know more about the people who were included in the study. This section uses data collected at Time One to summarise the age, gender and family circumstances of study participants. They have been divided into three groups in order to reflect the way in which location at the time of referral and assessment proved to be an important determinant of location at Time One.

In Table 3.1 the largest group – those who remained at home between their referral and the Time One interview and those who were discharged home from hospital – are shown in the first column. The second column refers to the group living at home at referral who were admitted to long-term care (abbreviated to LTC in the table). The third column includes those living in long-term care at referral and people who were assessed in hospital and discharged to long-term care.

There were twice as many women as men in the sample, a finding consistent with other samples of people using social services (Sinclair et al, 1990; Bowling et al, 1993).

At 84 (SD 6), the mean age of the women was slightly older than that of the men, whose mean age was 82 (SD 6), but this failed to reach significance (F=3.3; p=0.07). Consistent with the literature, the mean age of those living alone or in households of three or more people was greater than those living in two-person households (F=4.02; p=0.02). The explanation was that the two-person households usually consisted of the person with dementia and

Table 3.1: Characteristics of the older people by location from referral to Time One*

	% in the community and discharged home from hospital	% in the community admitted to LTC	% discharged from hospital to LTC and in LTC at referral	Valid *n*	Significance (2 df)
Age					NS
Less than 85	59	22	19	80	
85 and over	61	15	24	61	
Gender					NS
Men	61	18	21	44	
Women	59	19	22	97	
Social class					χ^2=7.4; *p*=0.02
I, II or III NM	82	10	8	38	
III M, IV or V	56	20	24	80	
Has a carer					χ^2=15.6; *p*=0.00
Yes	69	13	18	103	
No	34	37	29	38	
Sees relatives					NS
Yes	62	17	21	96	
No	41	29	30	34	
Sees friends					χ^2=10.1; *p*=0.006
Yes	72	9	19	54	
No	46	28	26	78	
% sample (*n*)	60 (84)	19 (27)	21 (30)	(141)	

*See glossary for explanation of significance. Percentages in this table and in all the tables and figures presented in the book may not total 100% due to rounding. Where the percentage sign is on the same line as the text, the table shows row percentages. Where it appears above the text, the table shows column percentages.

his or her spouse; people with dementia who are cared for by partners tend to be younger than those living alone or with others (Levin et al, 1989).

We were able to assign social class based on last known occupation of head of household to 85% of the older people. Where proxy informants were the chief source of information, it was less likely that we had sufficient data from which to assign social class.

The SSDs received referrals on behalf of people from all social classes during the study period, although the smaller numbers of people from social classes I and II mean that the categories have been collapsed in Table 3.1. The table suggests that people from social classes I to III non-manual were more likely to be living in the community at Time One, although this was not true of Time Two. The social class distribution among study participants was similar to that found in a representative sample of people with dementia living in the community (O'Connor et al, 1991).

Social class was strongly related to housing tenure, with three quarters of the people from social classes I and II being owner-occupiers, compared with half of those from social class III and a third of those from social classes IV and V (χ^2=8.4; 2 df; *p*=0.02). It is possible that considerations about housing equity may have delayed decisions to seek long-term care to some extent. This was certainly an issue for one carer.

"We will keep her in her own home for as long as possible, but fear that she will go into a home eventually and we will have nothing from it, so [my relatives] will have worked all their lives and the money will go on a residential home."

All but one of the older people were white, reflecting the ethnicity of all the referrals of people aged 65 and over to the social work teams during the study period (Moriarty and Webb, 1995). An SSI inspection of services for people with dementia also found very few people from black and Asian minority ethnic groups in their sample of active cases from eight SSDs (SSI, 1997). Why should this be the case?

One reason is the difference in demographic structure between the white and minority ethnic group populations in Britain. The 1991 Census data indicate that, overall, Britain's minority ethnic groups have a younger age structure than the white population (Warnes, 1996). Census data for the study areas showed that over 99% of the population aged 65 and over in the metropolitan borough and the county council were white; the corresponding figure for the London borough was 94%. However, this is set to change. While the proportion of people aged 74 and over who are from minority ethnic groups remains small, the Labour Force Survey showed that 13% of people describing their ethnic origin as Black-Caribbean and 7% of people describing their ethnic origin as Indian were aged 60-74; the proportion aged 60-74 in the white population was 14% (ONS, 1998). This means that SSDs can expect to see an increase in the number of referrals of older people from minority ethnic groups.

The second issue is whether older people from minority ethnic groups currently have fair access to health and social care services (Butt and Mirza, 1996). A study that used Family Health Services Authority records in order to examine the prevalence of dementia and depression among people from minority ethnic groups in Liverpool found that the number of people identified in this way was fewer than might have been expected on the basis of data from the Census. As we mentioned in Chapter 1, they found that many people from minority ethnic groups were either unaware of what help was available or felt that it was unsuitable (Boneham et al, 1997). The evidence suggests that, while this study was unable to offer insights into provision for people with dementia from minority ethnic groups, it is clearly a very important issue for the future (Patel, 1999; Patel et al, 1998).

Living arrangements and support

Household size and family support have been shown to be important factors in community service receipt and the likelihood of entry to long-term care (Levin et al, 1989; O'Connor et al, 1989b;

Sinclair et al, 1990; Wenger, 1994a). At the time of their referral, the overwhelming majority of study participants lived in private households, including the 19% (n=25) who lived in sheltered accommodation. This consisted mainly of local authority owned properties in the metropolitan borough. Just under 60% lived on their own and almost all the remainder lived with just one other person, usually their spouse. SSDs have traditionally had high numbers of people living alone among their clients and the proportion of people living alone was higher than that found in a community study (O'Connor et al, 1989b).

Overall, just under three quarters of the sample had a carer. This is a similar proportion to that found in a representative sample of frail older people (Buck et al, 1997). Table 3.1 shows that, in comparison with the other two groups, the majority of those who remained at home from referral until Time One and those who returned home from hospital had a carer. More information on the carers can be found in Chapter 5, while Chapter 7 explores the extent to which access to a carer determined whether or not the older people went into long-term care.

Wenger (1994b) has shown that people with dementia living in the community have higher levels of contact with relatives and lower levels of contact with friends, neighbours and community groups compared with older people who do not have dementia. At Time One, while 68% of the sample were reported to see a relative at least once a month, only 38% saw friends, and most of those in contact with friends were people living in the community. This is in keeping with other work, which has suggested that admission to long-term care reduces the range and type of social contacts of people with dementia (Myers and Seed, 1993).

Severity of dementia, depression and help received in completing ADLs

The instruments used to measure the presence of dementia, depression and functional disability are described in Chapter 2.

Of the 122 older people who were interviewed using the BAS (Macdonald et al, 1982), 43 were classified as having severe dementia; 75 scored between 3 and 7, and were classified as having mild or moderate dementia; four people scored below the cut-point for probable dementia. By Time Two, three of these four did score 3 or more, suggesting that they may have been mildly cognitively impaired at Time One. The fourth had died. She had been terminally ill at Time One and was depressed, as measured by her DEP score. It is possible that these factors may have affected her cognitive functioning when she was referred to the SSD. These four people have been excluded from subsequent analyses using the OBS dementia scores.

The proportion of people with severe dementia was higher than that in a study examining the prevalence of dementia in a sample derived from GP age–sex registers in Cambridge (O'Connor et al, 1989a). While we cannot exclude the possibility that this result can be attributed to our methods of sample selection, the evidence from other studies based on representative samples of people with dementia living in the community is that receipt of help from social services is linked with levels of functional disability (Livingston et al, 1990). This means that we would expect to find a higher proportion of people with severe dementia among SSD clients than in the overall population of people with dementia living in the community.

A third of the older people scored 7 or more on the DEP. This is the cut-off point shown to predict most accurately an independent rating of depressive symptoms by a psychiatrist in a sample of older people in residential homes (Mann et al, 1984). Only three people with severe dementia were able to answer at least one of the four filter questions, thereby completing the full BAS interview. This means that analyses comparing people with and without depression are almost exclusively based on people with mild to moderate dementia.

Having a carer, type of living arrangements, and contact with friends or relatives were not associated with depression, as measured by a score of between 7 and 28 on the DEP. However, almost half of the older people in long-term care at Time One scored 7 or more, compared with a fifth of those still living in the community (χ^2=5.54; 1 df; p=0.02). A few of the older people attributed feelings of sadness to their recent move into long-term care. Mrs Bruce confessed that:

"The bottom of it is that I don't like it here. I'd be lonely, I do feel lonely ... I wish I was in my own home."

The proportion of people in long-term care with depression is similar to that found in a study of admissions to local authority residential homes in London (Weyerer et al, 1995).

The mean number of ADL and IADL items with which participants received help from carers was three (SD 3) and four (SD 2), respectively. The equivalent figures in terms of help from services were five (SD 4) and three (SD 2). Help from services and from carers was strongly related to place of residence, with services providing more help to people in long-term care and carers providing more support to people in the community. This topic is discussed more fully in Chapters 5 and 7 in which we question whether the positive finding that carers would appear to receive more help with meeting the personal care needs of people with dementia than in the past can be offset against the wider picture that community services still appear to be unable to offer a level of support to people living in the community which matches that provided in long-term care.

Table 3.2 compares the three groups in terms of their mean scores on the DEP, the OBS and the number of ADLs with which they received assistance. The three groups differed in size, so it is important to treat differences in mean scores with caution. At Time One, people living in the community or discharged home from hospital had lower mean OBS scores than people who had been admitted to long-term care from the community. The mean number of ADLs with which they received assistance from services was lower in the community than in either of the two groups in long-term care but they received more assistance from carers.

Table 3.2: Depression, severity of dementia and assistance with ADLs by location from referral to Time One*

	In the community and discharged home from hospital	In the community admitted to LTC	Discharged from hospital to LTC and in LTC at referral	Valid n	Significance (2 df)
Mean DEP score (SD)	4 (4)	5 (4)	7 (5)	82	NS
Mean OBS score (SD)	6 (2)	7 (1)	7 (2)	118	F ratio=6.7; p=0.002
Mean n ADLs where services help (SD)	3 (3)	7 (3)	9 (2)	125	F ratio=68.8; p=0.000
Mean ADLs where carer helps (SD)	4 (3)	1 (2)	1 (2)	98	F ratio=10.5; p=0.001
Base n	84	27	30	141	

*See Chapter 2 for an explanation of how the BAS is administered. The four people scoring less than 3 on the OBS have been omitted from the OBS Scores but included in the DEP Scores. Scores range as follows: DEP, 0-24; OBS, 3-8; ADL assistance, 0-10. Integers have been rounded.

Changes in place of residence over the study period

One of the issues that emerged during the research was the difficulty in determining when changes, such as admissions to hospital, were temporary and when they signalled a permanent change in the life of the person concerned. Sometimes the answer became clear only after a few months. This is shown in Figure 3.2, which summarises some of the different pathways between community, hospital and long-term care settings. These various pathways are further illustrated in the series of case studies that follow.

The information in Tables 3.1 and 3.2 can be linked with that in Figure 3.2 and the case studies. The first column in Tables 3.1 and 3.2 relates to people living in the community and discharged home from hospital; in Figure 3.2 and the case studies they are represented by groups A and C. The second column in both tables represents group B, people who at referral were living in the community but who had been admitted to long-term care by Time One. The third column in the tables shows groups D and E, that is, those people who had been discharged to long-term care or were already living in long-term care when they were referred.

Figure 3.2 Pathways showing location between assessment and Time Two

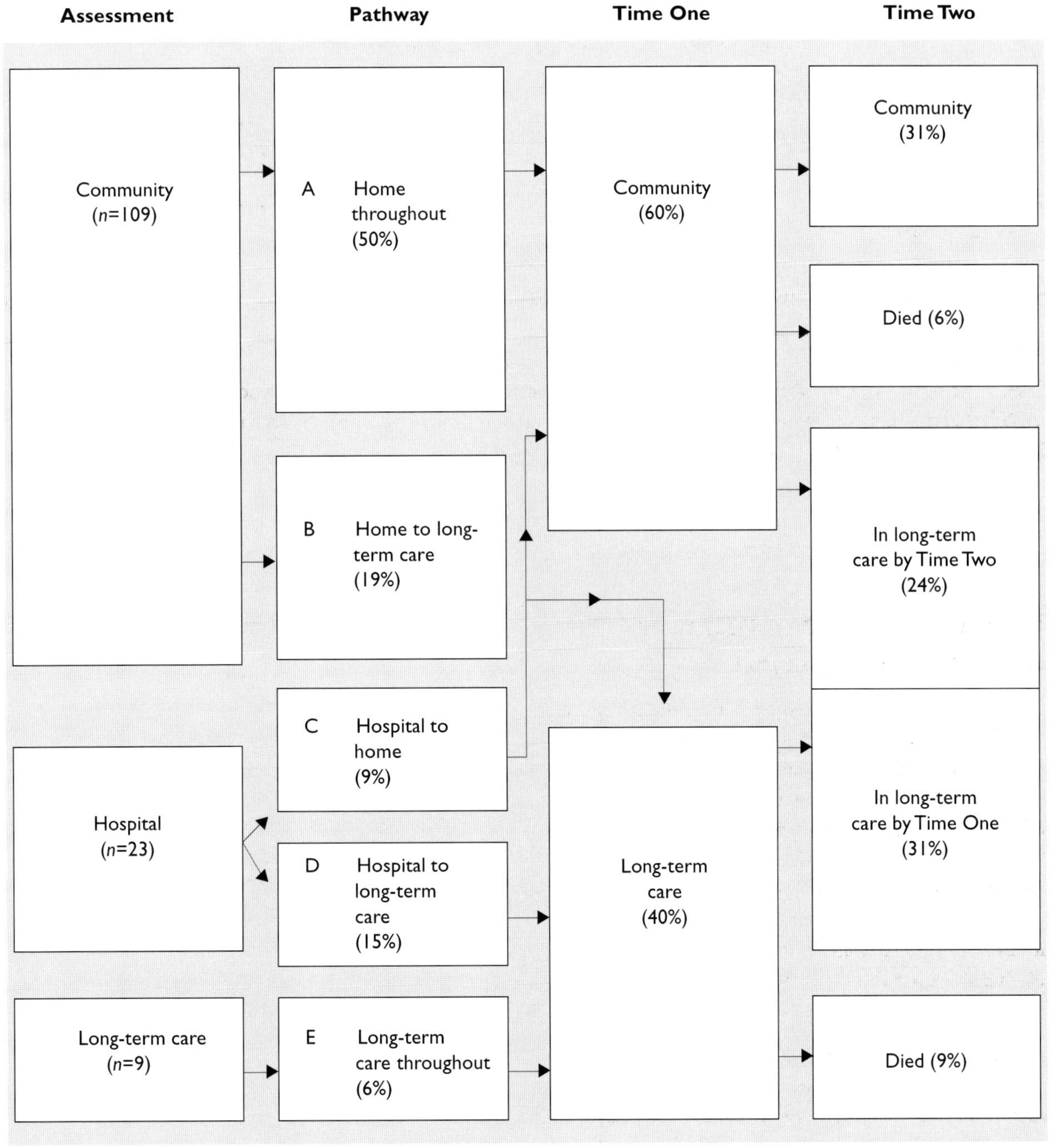

Figure shows column percentages

Group A: Home throughout

People in this group were more likely to have a carer.

> ## Case example
>
> Mr Simon cared for his wife with no services. Their son came to see them once a week but he did not provide any practical support. The couple were referred to the SSD by the CPN. The assessor suggested day care to Mr Simon. "[She] said she thought I needed a break." At Time One, Mr Simon said he wanted to "stay as we are for as long as possible. I can't see her happy in a home." By Time Two, Mrs Simon's memory was worse and Mr Simon explained that he could no longer leave her on her own. The Simons attended day care together twice a week. This gave Mr Simon a break from cooking and they both enjoyed the company. Mr Simon had also accepted the offer of a home-based carer support service so that he could attend a carers' group. He was finding caring increasingly difficult and was distressed that he found himself losing his temper with his wife more often. Nevertheless, he felt that the "only solution is to remain as we are, but I'd like a bit more help." He was particularly worried about what would happen if he was unable to continue caring for his wife.

Group B: From home to long-term care

These older people were more likely to live alone and less likely to have a carer.

> ## Case example
>
> Mrs Peters, a widow with no children, lived alone with no help other than that provided by her neighbour, Mrs Daniels. Mrs Peters was assessed after Mrs Daniels telephoned the SSD. "I wanted something done.... There wasn't the help there that was needed." Help was promised, but before anything could be arranged Mrs Peters fell and was admitted to hospital. Shortly after the Time One Interview, she was discharged to a nursing home where she died a few weeks later. Mrs Daniels felt cross and disappointed. "Mrs Peters worked hard all her life and when she needed help it wasn't there. She possibly could have stayed at home longer with extra help."

Group C: From hospital to home

Study participants who had been discharged home from hospital at Time One generally had co-resident carers (that is, carers who lived with the person for whom they cared). These older people were often in poor physical health.

> ## Case example
>
> Mr Phillips had spent five months in hospital for physical health problems. During his hospital stay, there was a marked deterioration in his levels of cognition. Mr and Mrs Phillips had never received any services and were reluctant to accept any help other than an hour of home care every morning to help Mr Phillips get up, wash and dress. Mrs Phillips rejected the idea of residential care for her husband. "If I can manage, it would be quite wrong." By Time Two, the amount of home care that they received remained unchanged but they had moved to a sheltered housing complex with a warden and alarm system. The highlight of their year had been a large family party. Mrs Phillips felt that she tended to become tired more easily, "but we can manage with help.... We want to stay together as we are."

Group D: From hospital to long-term care

People who were assessed in hospital and who went into long-term care tended to have severe dementia and to have lived alone before their admission. They included eight of the 11 people living in the community when they were referred who were subsequently admitted to hospital.

Case example

Mrs Kirk lived alone and had been receiving home care and meals-on-wheels for two years. Her daughter, Mrs Nicholas, was concerned about her well-being and contacted her mother's old age psychiatrist when her mother began to experience hallucinations. "She was in such a state, I thought she had to go somewhere." Mrs Kirk was admitted to hospital and the multidisciplinary team agreed that she should not return home but should move into a residential home. Mrs Nicholas was relieved. "I'm glad she is there – she couldn't possibly return home – but I do feel guilty in some ways because she didn't want to leave her home." At Time Two, while Mrs Nicholas remained concerned about her mother's changeable health, she was extremely pleased with the care that her mother had received. "They take everything off your shoulders and are very good."

Group E: Long-term care throughout

Generally, these referrals had been made because the older person's capital was running out or to request a transfer from residential to nursing care.

Case example

Mrs David had lived in a residential home for some years prior to the implementation of the 1990 NHS and Community Care Act. Her cognitive impairment was severe, but it was her level of physical disability that had led the home manager to request that she be assessed. She was admitted to hospital and it was agreed that she should be discharged to a local nursing home, where she died 18 months later.

Discussion

Comparisons of the demographic characteristics, severity of dementia and extent of family support highlighted the diversity among sample participants. The social class distribution and proportion of people with a carer was similar to that found in two studies based on representative samples derived from GPs' age sex–registers (O'Connor et al, 1989b, 1991; Buck et al, 1997), but higher proportions lived alone and had severe dementia. While the possibility of sample selection bias cannot be excluded, this is also likely to reflect underlying referral patterns to SSDs.

The number of referrals identifying issues associated with caring may reflect improved awareness of the needs of carers. While in some cases referrals were made on behalf of people with early dementia and they and their families may simply have needed information and advice, in many more instances the referral to the SSD came *after* a prolonged period of family care in which there had been no assistance from statutory services at all. There is evidence that caring has a 'wear and tear' effect (Knopman et al, 1988), and in these situations some carers will have reached a point at which they have decided that they do not wish to care any longer. When referrals are made in these circumstances, it is probable that community services are unlikely to enable continued residence in the community in the long-term. This is shown by the way in which some study participants moved to long-term care within a few months of the referral. In these cases information and advice will not be sufficient, and carers may need help in selecting a residential or nursing home and in coming to terms with their own feelings about ceasing to care.

A number of referrals occurred when temporary assistance was required, for instance where the carer had become ill or was away on holiday. Here, SSDs will need to consider what sort of help they are able to provide – is it to be in residential or nursing care, or are home care services able to take on the extent of additional support that would be required to substitute for the carer? The study data showed that people living in the community received more assistance with ADLs from carers than from services. It is not clear that current standard community provision has the capacity to take on the assistance provided by carers, even on a temporary basis.

At the same time, it should be appreciated that, numerically, referrals requiring temporary input made up a smaller proportion of overall referrals than those where carers sought long-term support, such as being provided with a regular break from caring. It is arguable that, if this long-term help is not provided, then temporary assistance will ultimately prove to be ineffective in sustaining carers looking after people with dementia in the community. Chapter 6 discusses the help that was provided regularly to people living in the community and their carers.

Proportionally few referrals were for cases that could be resolved quickly and closed. These included transfers from nursing to residential care or requests to take over the funding of long-term care. This indicates the long-term nature of the support that study participants, and other people with dementia in similar circumstances, would require. It has important implications for the way that care of people with dementia is managed, as we shall show in Chapter 7.

Although the number of referrals made by family members could be interpreted as a positive finding, reflecting better awareness of what SSDs have to offer, attention must be paid to ensuring that this improvement is consistent across all sections of the community. Nearly all the study participants and carers were white. As the proportion of older people from minority ethnic groups increases, SSDs must monitor that their referrals reflect this change. An SSI inspection of services to people from minority ethnic groups found examples of good practice, but also areas where improvements needed to be made (SSI, 1998b).

Those who entered long-term care relatively soon after referral were more likely to have severe dementia and less likely to have a carer. This is consistent with other research (Levin et al, 1989; Wenger, 1994b). It shows that good information on the severity of cognitive impairment and the extent and type of help provided by carers and other family members can be very useful in predicting where continued residence in the community can be supported and where long-term care is likely to be required.

An issue that became clearer as the study progressed was the way in which participants in the study moved between community, hospital and long-term care settings. This has methodological implications for future research. In order to reflect these transitions, we had to distinguish between the physical location of the person and his or her permanent residence. This was particularly apparent in cases where hospital admissions had occurred. In some cases the hospital stay was temporary and the older person returned home; in others it marked the stage between living at home and entering long-term care. More importantly, however, we must consider what effects such changes are likely to have on people with dementia. A number of people living in long-term care at Time One were depressed. As has been mentioned, they were less likely to have a carer. In addition, they were also less likely to see friends. The need to improve the process of transition to long-term care will be discussed further in Chapter 7.

Before we discuss in greater detail the receipt of services and what happened to people over the course of the study, we must return to events that occurred immediately after the referral. This is the topic of the following chapter, in which we discuss assessment.

Assessment

Key points

- This chapter reports on arrangements for assessment and review using information from assessors, carers, proxy informants and people with dementia.

- Most people were assessed shortly after being referred.

- Experiences of being assessed ranged from excellent to poor.

- People with dementia may find the process of being assessed stressful. This demands skill and sensitivity on the part of the assessor.

- Eighty-five per cent of assessments resulted in the provision of a new or increased service.

- Distinctions should be made between carers whose needs can be met by the assessment process itself and those who would benefit from continuing support.

Where it appears to the local authority that any person for whom they may provide or arrange for the provision of community care services may be in need of any such services, the authority –

(a)   shall carry out an assessment of his need for those services; and

(b)   having regard to the results of that assessment, shall then decide whether his needs call for the provision by them of any such services. (1990 NHS and Community Care Act, Section 47)

Introduction

Official documents had emphasised the importance of assessment in the successful implementation of the new arrangements. In readiness for the changes, the SSSI/SWSG had issued detailed practice guidance for both managers and practitioners (SSI/SWSG, 1991a, 1991b). This advised that:

- users and carers had information that would enable them to understand what was involved and what was likely to happen;

- assessments were based on need;

- users and carers should participate as fully as possible in the assessment process itself, and in any subsequent decisions about what help would be provided.

The way in which people with dementia are assessed has become a touchstone for some of the most important issues facing SSDs. First, there is the issue of risk. To what extent can the preferences of people with dementia be met without causing risk to them? Should risks to the carer's health outweigh the preferences of the person with dementia? Next is the degree to which other agencies are involved in the assessment process. People with dementia may have multiple needs, and so assessments are more likely to need the input of health and social services professionals. Then there is the question of arrangements for review. The needs of people with dementia will change over time. As we showed in Chapter 3, referrals were rarely related to problems that could be easily resolved. Finally, people with dementia remain one of the most under-represented groups in terms of being given an opportunity to comment on the services that they receive and in shaping future service delivery.

Variation in the way that assessments are completed

The need for greater consistency in social care is one of the major themes identified in the White Paper, *Modernising social services* (Secretary of State for Health, 1998). Hughes (1993) has suggested that there may be considerable variation in professionals' assessment standards. Writing prior to April 1993, she contrasted the localised and undisseminated examples of expertise and models of good practice in the assessment of older people with the widespread efforts to develop models of comprehensive assessment and multidisciplinary collaboration in respect of children and families. Assessors' professional backgrounds may influence the way in which they identify clients' needs (Rowlings, 1985; Taylor, 1993; Petch et al, 1994). Practitioners' levels of training and experience may influence the way they complete documentation (Parry-Jones and Caldock, 1995).

The format of assessment documentation also contributes to variation. The content of such documentation differs considerably between SSDs, with few assessment forms having being subjected to reliability or validity checks (Challis et al, 1996). There is no recommended standard set of assessment tools that reflect the objectives of the work of the personal social services (Nocon and Qureshi, 1996). This explains why there is now greater interest in finding standardised measures that are suitable for incorporating into SSD assessment proforma.

Obtaining users' and carers' perspectives on assessment

Although the views of younger people, especially those with mental health problems or physical disabilities, are receiving increasing and overdue attention, false assumptions may still be made about older people's willingness and ability to give their opinions (Thornton and Tozer, 1995). As Chapter 1 showed, the research base on the views of people with dementia is still limited (Stalker et al, 1999).

It is easier to ask about services received on a daily basis than one-off experiences that may have occurred some time ago. Tulle-Winton (1993) reported that around half of the 49 older people who were interviewed about their experiences of being assessed by a social worker had no recollection of either the visit or aspects of its content. Given that only "a few of the participants experienced a considerable degree of cognitive impairment" (sic), she questioned whether these results had occurred primarily because the older people did not view the assessment as an event that had relevance in their daily lives. By contrast, topics that *did* have relevance, such as their health or experience of home care, produced very good quality accounts. Thus, from the perspective of participants, being asked about assessments may be intrinsically less worthwhile than being asked about events in which they have a greater direct interest. This will be reflected in the data.

Hunter and colleagues (1993) suggest that one reason why greater reliance has been placed on assessment information collected from carers is that physical or mental incapacity among older users may mean that they are unable to be interviewed. To demonstrate this point, Hunter and colleagues had to exclude four of the 12 older people whom they had hoped to interview about their assessment. Unlike data for which there are 100% valid responses, where a considerable proportion of respondents have been unable to answer a question, the views expressed can never be presented as representative of the sample as a whole.

This helps explain why some studies have sought to examine users' experiences of the assessment process through observation (Caldock, 1992c; Meethan and Thompson, 1993).

How the study collected information on assessment

The approach we adopted was similar to that taken by Petch and colleagues (1996) in that we obtained information about the assessment from practitioners, users and carers.

Our first source of information was from interviews with the assessors (Moriarty and Webb, 1995). This produced quantitative data on the referral, assessment, referral source, the professionals undertaking the assessment and the services that they arranged as a result of the assessment. Assessors also provided their own perspective, explaining how they had approached the assessment and the key issues they had identified in drawing up the care plan.

Information from the assessors was given to the interviewers so that they would have background information before interviewing the carers. This was especially helpful when interviewing people whose first contact with the SSD was some time ago or those who had had multiple service contacts. It meant that carers and interviewers knew whether or not they were referring to the same event. Most of the questions used in interviewing the carers were open-ended.

At first, we thought that the proxy informants would also have information on the assessment. In the event, we found that they had generally neither been present nor had access to a record of what had happened. Many of the proxy informants were staff in long-term care settings who had not known the person with dementia before his or her admission, and they commented that they did not tend to receive information of this sort. Here, there is a dilemma between questions of confidentiality and the background information required in order to give good person-centred care. In Chapter 3, we reported on a similar dilemma when we explained that some proxy informants knew so little about the person with dementia's past life that we did not have

sufficient information from which to code social class. We wondered whether this was an unintended consequence of the separation of assessment from service provision.

Although a third of the older people had severe dementia, as measured by the OBS, about a fifth of those interviewed made some comment about the event.

To avoid problems with recall, Petch et al (1996) did not interview people who had been assessed more than three months before. The question of recall was also one that we had to consider, as the average time that had occurred since the assessment and the Time One interview was just over five months. However, many assessments were responses to specific events and, generally, these were still firmly at the forefront of carers' minds. Not enough is known about the circumstances in which people with dementia do remember details about the services that they receive. This means that we cannot comment on whether the interval between assessment and Time One did influence the proportion of people with dementia who were able to comment on the topic. However, it was considerably lower than the proportion able to comment on home care, day care and long-term care and was similar to the proportion who were able to remember a stay in short-term care.

Published information and waiting times for assessments

When the community care arrangements are fully in place local authorities will need to have in place published information accessible to all potential service users and carers ... setting out the types of community care services available, ... the assessment procedures to agree needs and ways of addressing them and the standards by which the care management system (including assessment) will be measured. (DoH, 1990, p 34)

Although it is not possible to make direct comparisons between pre- and post-April 1993 figures, research carried out before April 1993 suggested that it was unusual for families to get in touch directly with statutory services themselves (Sinclair et al, 1990). Almost a third of people included in the study had been referred to the SSD by their carer or another family member or friend (*n*=40) and one woman referred herself; 21% of the carers reported that they had decided to contact the SSD of their own volition, and a further 10% had done so at the suggestion of another family member.

In contrast with an earlier NISW study, in which carers sometimes referred to social workers as 'someone from the council' or the hospital (Levin et al, 1994), the carers were nearly all able to report that they knew the assessor's professional background or title. Some even produced business cards showing the assessor's name, telephone number and work base.

One of the main ways in which the government hopes to improve the way social services are delivered across authorities is through the publication of SSDs' annual performance records (DoH, 1999). The Audit Commission (1997) has reported that there is considerable variation in the time spent in completing assessments and arranging packages of care between authorities.

The interval between the date of the referral and the date of the assessment was calculated for 80% of the study participants. (Some assessment dates were missing from the assessor interview, either because the records were not readily available if the case was closed or because the informant was not the person who had completed the initial assessment.) Table 4.1 shows that the response time in the metropolitan borough was significantly quicker than in the others.

The mean interval of 19 days between referral and assessment is identical to the figure quoted by Petch and colleagues (1996) for assessments of older

people in four regions in Scotland. The range we found (0–130 days) was smaller than that in Scotland (0–168). In the study SSDs, 80% of assessments were completed within a month of the referral and it was exceptional for carers to report a delay in services being arranged.

The proposed Best Value Performance Indicators (BVPIs) suggest that the proportion of users and carers who said they got help quickly should be included as one of the BVPIs. We asked carers in the study their opinion of the time it had taken for the assessment. A third rated their SSD's response time as 'excellent' and half thought it 'very good'; only two people rated it as 'very poor'. Having collected information on response times in two ways, it seemed to us that the actual response time for assessments was a better measure of performance.

Involving carers in assessments

There was strong concordance between data from the assessor and carer interviews on whether or not the carer had participated in the assessment (κ=0.71).

Almost three quarters of the carers remembered being given a prearranged date and time for the assessment. There will always be circumstances in which this may not be possible. As we pointed out in Chapter 3, assessments sometimes took place in hospital in an emergency; other carers had long distances to travel or had paid employment commitments. However, 90% (*n*=68) of the carers who remembered being given notice of the assessment subsequently went on to attend it. Those who did not remember receiving advance notice of

Table 4.1: Waiting times for assessments

Study area	Mean number of days between referral and assessment (SD)	n	Significance
Metropolitan borough	12 (13)	43	
London borough*	26 (20)	25	
County	21 (19)	45	F=5.7; 2 df; p=0.004
Total	19 (18)	113	

*Our results for the London borough are almost identical to the ones reported for district and specialist teams in its 1995/96 community care plan. Equivalent information was not reported in those for the other two areas.

the assessment were unlikely to have been present (χ^2=38; 1 df; p=0.00). Six carers reported that they had not been given any feedback about the assessment whatsoever.

Involving people with dementia in assessments

Almost 70% of the carers who had attended the assessment reported that attempts had been made to seek the older person's views. This figure is likely to be an underestimate as their answers sometimes reflected their own perceptions of whether the person for whom they cared could express his or her opinions.

The uncertainty about the degree to which the person with dementia had been consulted during the assessment reflects the difficulties inherent in ensuring that they are able to make their views known. Official guidance increasingly recognises the role of advocacy for people with dementia as a means of supporting good practice in assessment and care management (Dunning, 1997). Although some SSDs have arranged for advocates to help clients being assessed (Knight, 1996), the advocacy schemes currently available for people with dementia have tended to be involved in representing the interests of people in long-term care or in a befriending capacity, rather than being directly involved in the assessment process.

In our study not a single person, whether carer or older person, was reported to have been accompanied at the assessment by anyone other than a family member or friend. According to the assessors, almost one in five of the older people (n=27) had been assessed alone; 12 of these people had no carer and in four cases the carer had ceased caring temporarily or permanently. By contrast, almost a fifth of carers reported that another member of their family or a friend had joined them in attending the assessment. This highlights the differing positions of study participants who could call upon family members for support and assistance during an assessment and those who could not.

Carers' experiences of assessment

In contrast to questions in which carers were asked to rate their satisfaction with the SSD and waiting times, their answers to the open-ended questions about the assessment produced a much wider range of responses. Analysis of the responses suggested that the content and standards of the assessment were very variable.

Case example

Mrs Benedict telephoned the SSD after her mother had fallen. "[The social worker] came out the next day.... He came and saw her here and discussed exactly what we needed to get her home.... [We] didn't fill in forms but [we tried] to work out what an ideal day would be for Mummy and then [tried] to arrange help for those things she couldn't do for herself.... Then [he] went to find out if he could get funding and then came back two days later. [We] signed [for] the care package and Mummy went home the next day."

Mrs Grant also looked after her mother, but her experience was quite different.

Case example

Mrs Grant telephoned the SSD because she was worried about her mother's deteriorating condition. "[The assessor] came to see me and Mum together and [he] said that she should have a home help. She refused at first but now accepts it. [He asked questions] about her condition. [There was] lots of form filling. [My mum] was a bit on her guard, she was very mixed up. She couldn't remember my name or my sister's name.... The home care organiser] then came and she was still refusing any help ... but I pressed the subject.... [I] think that you need to be with the person being assessed for quite a while to see what they are really like."

This was a recurrent response pattern. Some carers reported that the assessment was dominated by the need to fill in forms; others that there were none. Some felt that their views had been listened to and all the alternatives explained; others that the process was too rushed. The negotiation skills of some workers were questioned by some; others had nothing but admiration for their assessor:

> "Robert had a very careful, casual approach.... There were no forms at all. [My husband was] worried at first. [He] doesn't know anything is wrong with him but Robert made the effort to gain his trust. [Robert] kept chatting. He avoided direct questions – [it was] a deliberate ploy."

The variability of the responses suggested that experiences of assessment varied within teams, within types of teams and within areas, but that, taken together, those carers whose accounts suggested that time had been taken to find out how they were coping and whether they needed help were most likely to report that they were satisfied with the assessment (χ^2=13.5; 2 df; p=0.001).

Views of people with dementia about assessment

While proportionally fewer of the people with dementia could remember the assessment in any detail, those that did were able to speak movingly and clearly about how they had felt. Mrs Charles remembered feeling very concerned about the potential consequences of being assessed:

> "[I was] not happy. [I was] quite cross and miserable – I thought she [social worker] wanted to put me in a home."

Others found that it was process of being assessed that had made them feel anxious. One of these was Mrs Edwards:

> "[The social worker] asked routine questions. Was I being looked after? Did I need any help? [I felt] a bit jittery at first. What now? What will he ask? He did say something [about arranging more help] but I don't like strange people – I'd sooner do my own things."

Some assessments had occurred at times of crisis or change in people's lives. Mr Neill had been referred to the SSD when his former partner decided to move away and give up any involvement in his care. Perhaps this was what he was recalling when he mentioned:

> "In actual fact, the way she [social worker] came to it didn't please me very much. It was coupled up with something I didn't like."

These comments serve to emphasise the skills needed in assessing people with dementia.

Negotiating between users and carers

One of the most difficult roles for assessors is in balancing the needs and preferences of people with dementia with those of their carers. It was Twigg (1988) who first raised the issue of the ambiguous position held by carers within the social care system, in which carers can be seen as providers of care or as co-clients. Clarke and colleagues (1993) have suggested that, if carers' mental or physical health appears to be affected, then professionals view the carer as client, rather than the person being cared for. Myers and MacDonald (1996) have suggested that:

> The power of carers may therefore derive from the 'service' they offer and the potential threat of 'withdrawal' from that service. In other words, it is their power of exit as providers. (Myers and MacDonald, 1996, p 93)

The example of Mrs Henry demonstrates this point well.

Case example

Since the death of his wife 20 years before, Mrs Henry had looked after her cousin, Mr Gregg, by cooking his meals, doing his washing and so on. Three years before, Mr Gregg had been diagnosed as having Alzheimer's Disease. The district nurse made the referral to the SSD on behalf of Mrs Henry. "I refused to look after him any more. They'd got to find somebody to do it because there was nobody else and waiting lists all over the place – I'd tried to get meals on wheels but [there was a] waiting list."

In other cases, it was the carer who tried to ensure that the wishes of the person with dementia were respected, despite the risks involved. The following example illustrates the difficulties in balancing professional judgements against the preferences of an individual.

Case example

Mr Julian had looked after his mother for two years since noticing that she had problems with her memory. She had refused previous offers of services and was eventually admitted to hospital where she was assessed. Mr Julian attended the ward meeting to discuss what should happen. "They said that a residential home would be best but I said that my mother wouldn't want this so I found her the warden controlled flat and she went there." The social worker involved in the assessment gave her view: "The recommendation of the multidisciplinary team was that Mrs Julian needed long-term care but the family were put out by this and arranged for her to move into warden controlled accommodation – it's a lovely flat. We agreed to see how it went with a package of care on a trial basis but she's doing much better than the team thought she would." Shortly afterwards, Mrs Julian's mental state meant that she could no longer be cared for in sheltered housing and she was admitted to a nursing home.

Involving other agencies in assessments

The 1990 NHS and Community Care Act specified that SSDs might need to involve other agencies, such as health and housing, in assessments. On the basis of information from the assessors, just under half of the assessments overall and 40% of assessments of people with carers had involved consultation with another professional. A third of these assessments had involved discussions with more than one professional. This is similar to the picture reported in Petch and colleagues (1996), where 52% of older people in the case sample were reported to have received a specialist assessment by

medical or nursing staff or staff in professions allied to medicine in addition to that completed by the practitioner in the social work department. In our study, the professionals most frequently mentioned as having been involved in the process were old age psychiatrists ($n=18$) and ward or day hospital nursing staff ($n=13$).

About a third of all the assessments and three quarters of those in which consultation with another professional took place ($n=49$) resulted in a joint assessment in which the SSD assessor, other professional(s) and the older person all met together. This was most likely to occur in assessments completed by hospital social work teams ($\chi^2=9.85$; 2 df; $p=0.01$). Once more, ward and day hospital staff and old age psychiatrists were the most frequently mentioned professional grouping, suggesting that logistical considerations may have played a role in facilitating joint assessments.

When several professionals or agencies are involved in an assessment, it raises issues about who should take responsibility for coordinating and passing on information to all those who are involved. As well as asking the assessors about contact with other professionals, we also asked the carers who had attended the assessment meetings and whether the person with dementia had received any other assessments. While we cannot discount the possibility of recall bias, the concordance between the carers' and social workers' reports on which other professionals had been involved in the assessment was relatively low ($\kappa=0.48$). It appeared to reflect a tendency both for some carers to include additional contacts other than those defined by the social worker as having been part of the assessment process, and for details of assessor contacts with other professionals outside the assessment meeting not always to have been passed on to the carers.

The extent to which assessments by different professionals might duplicate each other has also been raised (SSI, 1996; Audit Commission, 1997). For example, the SSI suggested that:

Few systems exist for joint referral or joint response. Those older people with dementia who are identified as at risk will be likely to receive multiple unrelated assessments and care plans from a variety of professionals. (SSI, 1996, p 7)

The study collected information on the assessment from SSD assessors, carers and proxy informants but not from other professionals. This means that we cannot comment on the extent to which the social worker's assessments duplicated those completed by others. However, some carers did raise this as an issue. Mrs Stanley, who looked after her father-in-law, pointed out the need for improved coordination:

> "A district nurse came and we didn't know and no one [ie other than Mr Stanley] was in ... [Assessor] came again and arranged day care so that [Mr Stanley] could be assessed. We were all most upset at how he was assessed – he was sent from one [day centre] to another. They just wanted to shuffle him about."

While there are potential conflicts with a person with dementia's rights to confidentiality, there is scope for greater clarity about the circumstances in which information about the assessment is shared. Given that so few proxy informants had been present for the assessment (just four out of 30, excluding two cases where the assessor was the proxy informant and two non-professional proxy informants), it would appear that this is an issue about sharing information not just with carers but also with service providers. Mrs Lyle, a warden who acted as a proxy informant, regretted the lack of opportunity for joint discussion:

> "I do feel there should be more feedback from social services to wardens. I don't feel we are regarded as [if we are] as 'professional' as other bodies. At the end of the day, we have first hand contact and experience with the clients. We get to know them but we are not asked to get involved."

Assessing carers' needs

The need to make practical support for carers a high priority was one of the six key objectives of the reforms outlined in *Caring for people* (Secretaries of State, Health, Social Security, Wales and Scotland, 1989). The theme was continued with the publication of *Modernising social services* (Secretary of

State for Health, 1998). The Time One interviews took place before the 1995 Carers (Recognition and Services) Act was implemented. At this time, few carers reported that they had either heard of or been offered a separate assessment of their needs. By Time Two, 19% ($n=17$) of the carers who were re-interviewed said that they had heard of the Act, but no one said that they had asked to be assessed themselves. It is unlikely that these levels of awareness are atypical. Most carers who had heard of the legislation said that they learnt of it through the media or their membership of the Carers National Association (CNA) or Alzheimer's Society. One carer said that a social worker had come to his carers' group in order to talk to members about the Act.

However, it would be mistaken to assume that the lack of carer assessments indicated that no account was taken of carers' needs. Sixty per cent of the carers made comments suggesting that some attention had been made to incorporating their views or providing support for them. One of these was Mrs Walter, whose GP had referred her to the SSD:

> "Jackie's [assessor] very nice.... She said she would arrange for him to go to [day care] and now she's arranged an extra day.... I just tell her how he's going on and she tells me what to expect.... She says 'if you've got any problems, if you feel like going out and screaming, just give me a ring'.... John [husband] likes her – he's seen her at [day care]."

Once more, the variation in practice was a recurring theme. Mrs Oswald's experiences were different from Mrs Walters':

> "I was having the worst time I'd ever had.... [Assessor] came and thought I could manage with [help with shopping]... I wasn't aware that it was an assessment – I was more or less told that I could manage."

Her reply to the question on the advice that she would give to someone else in her position who was thinking of getting in touch with the SSD was laconic:

> "The best of British!"

However, there was evidence that continued contact, as measured by whether the carer had seen the assessor since the assessment, the number of times the assessor had been seen and whether a future appointment had been arranged, was being focused on carers who seemed to be experiencing more difficulties. The mean GHQ scores of carers who had received greater social work input was higher than those of carers who had not ($F=8.12$; 1 df; $p=0.0001$). This suggests that, in their assessments, the social workers may have identified carers who were in poorer psychological health and continued to give them support. However, there were a number of carers who would have wanted social work support but did not receive it.

Service provision as a result of the assessment

Eighty-five per cent of assessments resulted in the provision of a new or increased service. This was most usually home care and day care (see Chapter 6) or the offer of a place in long-term care (see Chapter 7). The finding that assessments did result in changes to the service received is important. It has been suggested that if GPs perceive services to be unavailable this may influence whether they take the step of referring a person to the SSD (Iliffe et al, 1994). Equally, the referrer needs to be notified of any changes. The level of feedback SSDs give to GPs has been found to be variable (Lloyd et al, 1995). This may also have the effect of reducing referral rates (SSI, 1996).

Review arrangements

The White Paper *Modernising social services* (Secretary of State for Health, 1998) has outlined that action will be taken to improve review and follow-up arrangements in order to take account of people's changing needs. Nearly 40% ($n=32$) of the carers re-interviewed said that they were familiar with the term 'review'. Reflecting the fact that so many of the sample were now in long-term care, the same proportion said that they would be most likely to contact staff in residential or nursing homes in order to discuss how the person with dementia was getting on; 21% ($n=18$) said that they would get in

touch with the social worker and 14% ($n=12$) with the GP.

In contrast to their knowledge of the assessment, with which they were rarely directly involved, the proxy informants were more likely to know about review arrangements for the older people. This was because many of them were staff working in long-term care who had actually participated in review meetings.

On the basis of information from the carers and proxy informants, two thirds ($n=69$) of the people in the sample who were still alive and who were re-interviewed had seen the original assessor or another social worker in the 11 months or so between Times One and Two. Within this, there was a wide range of contact; some older people had been seen just once, others every one or two months. A third of the older people who had been reviewed were reported to have been given either a definite or a provisional date for their next appointment. This raises issues about the lack of clarity about what constitutes good practice in review arrangements, which are discussed more fully in Chapter 7.

Almost three quarters of the people living at home at Time Two ($n=25$) had seen the assessor or another social worker. Of the 11 who had not, two had seen a home care organiser and four had been contacted by telephone. Excluding those who had died, two thirds of the people in long-term care were reported to have been reviewed. While it is customary to close cases of self-funding residents assessed by the SSD once they have settled, some of the people who were reported not to have had contact with the assessor or another social worker were funded by the SSD. It is possible that their care had been reviewed but that this information had not been passed on to their carers.

Discussion

Although the skills and processes needed to undertake assessment and desired outcomes for users are broadly similar for all user groups, the nature of dementia requires special skills if quality assessments of older people with dementia are to be achieved. (SSI, 1996, p 15)

Our findings suggested that the arrangements for assessment within the study areas showed features that were both encouraging and less favourable. The most notable feature was the high number of assessments that had resulted in the provision of a new or increased service. The proportion of carers (a third) who reported that they had contacted the SSD themselves suggests an improved awareness of potential sources of help. In the same way, most carers were aware of the name and professional background of the assessor and where he or she was based. Nevertheless, distinctions must be made between this type of knowledge and the sort that enables users and carers to make informed comparisons between different types of service.

Although this study did not find any examples of assessments where advocates were present, this is likely to be an issue for the future. Many people with dementia have the capacity to put their views forward and have carers and other family members who are prepared to support them in achieving what they want from the assessment. However, this presents a sharp contrast with the case of people with severe dementia who do not have any family.

Although increasing emphasis is being given to finding ways of monitoring the performance of SSDs, there are questions about the extent to which monitoring systems for all adult clients are suited to measuring the quality of their services for people with dementia. For instance, it has been suggested that providing an effective service to people with dementia in the community requires a more intensive system than periodic reviews (Sturges, 1997). This raises the question of how SSDs integrate performance assessment measurement systems for people with dementia with those for other client groups.

At the same time, the comments of the older people and carers suggested that the way in which they measured their satisfaction with the assessment was not simply a question of issues such as waiting times, but lay in satisfaction with the practice and interpersonal skills of the assessors themselves. When assessors built up a relationship of trust, explained options and took account of the views of the user and carer, it was time that was well spent. Equally, the negative experiences reported by some study participants suggests that more work is needed on identifying the practice skills required in order to assess effectively and sensitively. Skill is required in identifying risk, in negotiating between people with dementia and their carers, in giving information on a range of service options, and in helping people make emotionally difficult transitions, such as moving to long-term care. These are some of the dilemmas discussed in the next chapter, which looks at the position of carers in more detail.

Responding to the needs of carers

Key points

- **This chapter describes the carers in the sample and examines their sources of advice and support.**

- **Compared with services and other family members, carers were providing most practical help for people living in the community.**

- **More recognition should be given to the distinct needs of different types of carer.**

- **Carers under retirement age were often combining their caring responsibilities with full or part-time paid employment.**

- **Current co-resident carers, who were mainly spouses, cared for people with more severe dementia, provided most assistance and appeared to be at greatest risk of poor psychological health.**

- **The information needs of carers were not always met.**

"Last time you came, you kept on referring to me as a carer. I didn't know what you meant. Then I thought about it and I thought you must think I'm a bit slow!"
(Mr Norman, interviewed at Time Two)

Introduction

Studies of older people have repeatedly shown that their lives cannot be considered in isolation from those of their families (Phillipson, 1992). In Chapters 2 and 3, we explained that almost three quarters of people with dementia in our study had an identified carer. As we followed through events in the lives of study participants, we also had to consider their significance for the carers.

There are many reviews of the literature on caregiving (Parker, 1990; Twigg et al, 1990; Twigg and Atkin, 1994; Manthorpe, 1994; Nocon and Qureshi, 1996; Levin, 1997; Moriarty, 1998). Instead of describing results from the study that replicate those to be found elsewhere, we shall concentrate on those findings that highlight most clearly the support from health and social services that carers in the study received following the implementation of the 1990 NHS and Community Care Act.

Helping carers is one of the best ways of helping the people they are caring for. Help for carers cannot be seen in isolation from help for the person for whom they are caring. Providers of the range of services and benefits which exist to meet the needs of sick, disabled or frail elderly people must recognise that the patient or user of services and their carer are closely linked, and must not neglect the carer's existence and needs.
(Her Majesty's Government, 1999, p 12)

In this chapter we shall examine support in the form of advice and information and support from professionals. We shall also consider the carers' sources of support from within their circle of family and friends. This will set the background for the following chapter, in which we discuss practical help in the form of services.

Types of carer included in the study

Carers were defined as anyone giving unpaid assistance with one or more ADLs or IADLs at least once a week at the time of referral. Interviews took place with three types of carer:

i) About a third of the carers ceased to care for someone living in the community in the six-month interval between referral and Time One. We called these '*former*' carers, although only six of the 32 carers in this group were no longer giving any weekly assistance with ADLs or IADLs by Time One.

ii) Among those who had continued to care for someone living in the community at Time One, proportionally more people cared for someone who did not live in their household. They are described as '*non-resident carers*'.

iii) Carers who lived in the same household at Time One as the person for whom they cared are referred to as '*co-resident carers*'.

Previous research has shown how important it is to distinguish between co-resident and non-resident carers, because the two groups tend to differ both in terms of their relationship to the person for whom

Table 5.1: Characteristics of the carers*

	% current co-resident carers	% current non-resident carers	% former carers	Valid *n*	Significance
Gender					NS
Men	29	40	31	35	
Women	30	40	30	67	
Relationship to older person					$\chi^2=60; p=0.00$
Spouse	76	-	24	34	
Daughter	7	59	34	29	
Other	5	62	33	39	
Age					$\chi^2=35; p=0.00$
Less than 65	7	60	33	58	
65 and over	58	14	28	43	
In paid employment					$\chi^2=21; p=0.00$
Yes	3	64	33	36	
No	44	27	29	66	
Annual income					$\chi^2=12; p=0.02$
Up to £9,999	44	29	27	52	
£10,000 and above	10	53	37	38	
Social class					NS
I, II or III NM	25	47	28	53	
III M, IV, or V	34	33	33	40	
% sample (*n*)	30 *(30)*	40 *(41)*	30 *(31)*	*(102)*	

*In Chapter 2 we explained that two of the older people were cared for by the same person who acted as a double informant. This means that in this chapter tables presenting characteristics of the carers show data for 102 individuals but those presenting characteristics of the older people with carers have a base of 103.

they care and in the amount of assistance that they give (Arber and Ginn, 1991; Parker and Lawton, 1994; Wenger, 1990).

Demographic characteristics of the carers

The contrasts between current co-resident and non-resident carers are shown clearly in Table 5.1, which summarises some of the main characteristics of the carers who were interviewed.

The ratio of women to men carers was 2:1. Overall, 89% of carers were married. Their mean age was 63 (SD 13). All but one described themselves as white. These characteristics are very similar to those interviewed as supporters of confused older people living in the community in the first NISW dementia study (Levin et al, 1989).

Consistent with the literature, the carers were predominantly the older people's spouses and adult children. Other kin included siblings, cousins, nieces and nephews. The only non-kin current carer described herself as a family friend.

The majority of co-resident carers were married to the person for whom they cared (spouse carers). By contrast, non-resident carers were generally caring for a parent. This explains why they tended to be younger than co-resident carers and why they were more likely to be in paid employment. The proportion of men and women carers below retirement age who worked outside the home was very similar, with just over two thirds of carers being in paid employment. This is in keeping with the increasing participation of women in the labour force within society as a whole. Men carers under the age of retirement who had stopped working usually described themselves as not being in paid employment because of ill-health. In contrast, just under half of the women under retirement age who were not in paid employment attributed it to their caring responsibilities or other family commitments.

As most co-resident carers were over the age of retirement, it was not surprising that their annual income was lower that that of non-resident carers. Just under half of the carers aged 65 and over (*n*=17) received an occupational pension but only

five had an occupational pension large enough to take their annual income into the £10,000-and-over bracket when it was combined with their state pension and other sources of income.

Forty per cent of the older people living at home at Time One received Attendance Allowance or Disability Living Allowance at the higher rate, and another 40% received it at the lower rate. However, only three carers received Invalid Care Allowance (ICA). In fact, there was only one other carer under retirement age whose income level suggested that she would have qualified for ICA, but she did not care for 35 hours per week so the low levels of receipt would not seem to be explained by poor uptake of the benefit. Rather, the low earnings limit, the age restriction on ICA and its effect on the receipt of other benefits means that, while many carers of people with dementia are giving substantial amounts of care, their contribution is not recognised by the current state benefits system.

There has been little research focusing on social class and caring. Secondary analysis of data from the 1985 GHS found that carers living in households from the skilled manual, semi-skilled and unskilled classes were more likely to provide co-resident care than those from the higher and lower middle classes (Arber and Ginn, 1992). We found the same pattern of social class and co-residence.

It was striking that the distribution of social class of carer, based on occupation or last occupation of the head of household, differed from that of the older people themselves (reported in Chapter 3). A higher proportion of carers (30%) came from social classes I and II in comparison with 20% of the older people.

Taking on caring responsibilities

Carers had started to provide support under a range of circumstances. Sometimes they had gradually begun to give more and more help to the older person. Mrs Douglas explained:

"I've always cared for him as a wife, but fifteen years ago I noticed he was slower and things have gradually got worse."

Others could date their involvement from a specific event, for example after the older person was admitted to hospital or after a decrease in his or her support network. Many of the carers who were adult children reported that the death of one parent had meant that they had to undertake his or her role in supporting the surviving partner. Mrs Oliver's mother-in-law had developed cognitive impairment shortly before her referral to the SSD. However, it was the preceding 12 years of care that had followed her father-in-law's death that were, in Mrs Oliver's opinion, responsible for the current tension in her marriage.

"She was OK for about six months after her husband died and then it was a question of Andrew [son], correction me, [doing it] – 'You're his wife. You should look after me.... If she wasn't in [long-term care] now, I probably would have left my husband."

According to the carers, the older people had shown problems with short-term memory or other signs of cognitive impairment for an average of four years before the Time One interview. The older people who had experienced memory problems longest were those with current co-resident carers (5 years, SD 4) compared with those with non-resident carers (3 years, SD 2) (F-ratio=3.6; p=0.03). This is supported by the evidence from the OBS scores (Macdonald et al, 1982), which showed that there were proportionally more people with mild or moderate dementia living alone. Another factor possibly contributing to the difference between the groups is that memory deficits tend to become apparent sooner when the person affected lives in a household with other people.

Forty-three per cent of the carers reported that they had taken on a caring role prior to observing short-term memory problems or other signs of cognitive impairment in the older person, so the length of time for which they had cared did not always coincide with the onset of cognitive impairment in the older person. At Time One, on average, they had been caring for six years (SD 7). However, former carers reported that they had been assisting the person for whom they cared for an average of eight and a half years, compared with five years for current co-resident and non-resident carers (t=-2.3; p=0.03). This raises the question of whether caring has a 'wear and tear' effect, in which carers' capacity

to undertake a caring role is gradually worn away (Silliman, 1993). It may also suggest that care needs which predate and are additional to those posed by dementia, such as a physical disability, may combine to increase the risk of entry to long-term care for the person with dementia (Reddy and Pitt, 1993).

Visits to the person with dementia

Chapter 2 described the extent of contact between carers and the people with dementia. Non-resident carers visited an average of eight times a week (SD 9). The range was 1-42, showing that some carers were making two or three visits per day. On average, former carers were visiting three times (SD 3) per week.

It was much more usual for non-resident carers to visit the older person than the reverse. Unsurprisingly, the number of visits that they made was associated with the length of the journey between their homes and those of the older people. On average, carers with a journey time of less than a quarter of an hour visited eight times a week. Those whose journeys lasted 15-29 minutes or 30-59 minutes visited twice a week and carers with a journey time of over an hour visited once a week. The carers who were most likely to visit at least once a day were those who lived within walking distance of the person with dementia (F=4.4; p=0.03). Excluding these carers, most non-resident carers made their journeys by car.

However, access to a car was less usual among some of the former carers, particularly those who were spouses. Mr Rogers liked to visit his wife every day. He had problems walking and needed to take a taxi to the residential home in which she lived. His net weekly income was £69 and he paid £3 each way for a taxi ride. When asked about his financial circumstances, he replied:

"It's going worse and worse. [My problems] are only my money troubles. After the bills, there's not much left, is there? There's no chance you can manage."

Mrs Trevor had also experienced this problem. When her mother moved into long-term care, her father was still living at home.

"We got very good backup from social services but I feel more should be done to ensure couples should be together.... In my father's case, it's often difficult to get to visit mum and mostly he has to rely on family to get him there.... When a couple have been together 60 years, it seems cruel that they cannot always spend their last years together."

Assistance given by co-resident and non-resident carers

Table 5.2 shows that co-resident carers were looking after people with more severe dementia, as measured by the OBS (Macdonald et al, 1982), and that they provided greater assistance with ADLs and IADLs. However, they were less likely to be supported in these activities by others such as other family members.

The low number of IADLs with which services assisted may reflect the wider shift towards providing personal care at the expense of household tasks, such as shopping or cleaning. This is discussed more fully in Chapter 6. It is possible to argue that the similarity between ADL assistance to people with co-resident and non-resident carers reflects a

positive move away from the tendency to provide home care services to people living alone at the expense of people with similar needs who have co-resident carers.

Carers' psychological health

The psychological consequences of caring have been well documented. There is some evidence suggesting that carers for people with dementia report greater strain, and experience greater psychological morbidity, than carers for other older people (O'Connor et al, 1990; Livingston et al, 1996; Wijeratne and Lovestone, 1996).

Overall, 37% of the carers scored six or higher on the GHQ-28 at Time One, the cut-point that we used to denote scores suggesting that they were likely to be experiencing symptoms associated with psychiatric illnesses such as depression and anxiety (Goldberg and Williams, 1988). As she completed the GHQ, Mrs Hugo, who cared for her mother in law, exclaimed:

"I've never had these feelings before. Are my next 20 years going to be like this?"

Table 5.2: Characteristics of the people with current co-resident and non-resident carers, and the help provided to them by carers, services and others*

	People with co-resident carers (SD)	People with non-resident carers (SD)	Valid *n*	Significance
Mean OBS score	7 (2)	6 (2)	58	*t*=2.6; *p*=0.01
Mean DEP score	3 (3)	4 (3)	42	NS
Mean *n* ADLs in which carer helps	5 (3)	3 (2)	66	*t*=4.4; *p*=0.000
Mean *n* IADLs in which carer helps	5 (1)	4 (2)	62	*t*=3.3; *p*=0.002
Mean *n* ADLs in which services help	3 (3)	2 (2)	62	NS
Mean *n* IADLs in which services help	1 (1)	2 (1)	57	*t*=-2.2; *p*=0.04
Mean *n* ADLs in which others help	<1 (1)	2 (2)	56	*t*=-3.3; *p*=0.002
Mean *n* IADLs in which others help	1 (1)	3 (2)	53	*t*=-4.6; *p*=0.000
Base *n*	30	41	71	

*Scores on the OBS range, 0-8; the DEP, 0-24; ADLs, 0-10; IADLs, 0-6. All mean scores and standard deviations have been rounded to integers.

The proportion of carers scoring six or higher on the GHQ-28 is very similar to that found in earlier NISW studies using services samples (Levin et al, 1989, 1994) but is higher than one might expect to find in a random sample of the general population (Bowling et al, 1992).

The carers were asked about their self-rated health and the presence of a limiting long-standing illness or disability using the questions used in the GHS. Carers aged 65 and over were more likely to rate their health as poor and to report that they had a long-standing illness or disability.

Information on life events was collected by asking two questions: 'Has anything particularly upsetting happened to you or a member of your family over the last year?' and 'Has anything particularly

enjoyable happened?' (Brown, 1974). We included life events in these categories only if we judged them to be 'independent' of the older person and the caring situation (for instance, the death of another family member).

Table 5.3 shows that scores of six or higher on the GHQ-28 at Time One were associated with poor self-reported health, having a limiting long-standing illness and experiencing an upsetting life event.

As we explained earlier, there were more co-resident carers among people from social classes III M, IV or V. The association between high GHQ-28 scores and membership of these social classes is likely to be explained by the higher prevalence of spouse carers in this group.

Table 5.3: Factors associated with high GHQ scores (all carers)

	% scoring 0-5 on the GHQ-28	% scoring 6-28 on the GHQ-28	Valid *n*	Significance
Gender				NS
Men	70	30	33	
Women	56	44	65	
Currently caring				NS
Yes	61	39	67	
No	61	39	31	
Self-rated health				$\chi^2=14.3; p=0.001$
Good	83	17	40	
Fairly good	52	48	29	
Not good	39	61	28	
Long-standing illness or disability				$\chi^2=11.7; p=0.001$
Yes	42	58	43	
No	76	24	54	
Upsetting life event				$\chi^2=5.6; p=0.02$
Yes	46	54	37	
No	70	30	60	
Carer's social class				$\chi^2=7.5; p=0.006$
I, II or III NM	74	26	50	
III M, IV, or V	47	53	47	
Relationship to person cared for				$\chi^2=6.7; p=0.03$
Spouse	50	50	30	
Daughter	52	48	29	
Other	77	23	39	
% sample (*n*)	61 (60)	39 (38)	98	

Carers also answered a series of questions about the older person's behaviour, including 'trying behaviours' (such as repeating the same question or action over and over), sleep disturbance and aggression, and they reported on positive personality traits (such as showing affection and appreciation) (Levin et al, 1989). (The full list is included in Appendix 3.) Carers with high GHQ-28 scores were more likely to be looking after someone with more reported trying behaviours (t=-3.4; p=0.001) and fewer positive traits (t=3.0; p=0.003).

The finding that spouses and daughters were at particular risk of scoring highly on the GHQ-28 is consistent with the literature. It is likely to reflect a greater caring input and, in the case of spouses, to be accentuated by the likelihood of poorer physical health, than for other types of carer.

Information needs

The provision of information, advice and counselling are key requirements for carers of older people with dementia (Levin et al, 1989; Marshall, 1997). The study found that carers wanted two types of information. First, they wanted to be told about the diagnosis and prognosis of their relatives' problems. Mrs Roberts, who cared for her mother, explained:

"It would be helpful if someone would tell us what to do, how to cope with the situation. If someone would tell us what is the matter with her. We suspect she has senile dementia; no one has ever told us."

This is consistent with other research suggesting that most carers would want to know the diagnosis of a family member with Alzheimer's Disease and that a substantial proportion would consider predictive testing were it available (Maguire et al, 1996).

Carers were asked whether they had been given a name for the older person's problems. Just over a third of the carers said that they had been told that the older person had Alzheimer's Disease or another specific dementia sub-type: 30% spoke of 'dementia'; the remainder mentioned symptoms such as confusion or attributed the older person's problems

to his or her physical health. Mrs Thomas, caring for her non-resident mother, said:

"The GP just says 'confused'. She's never explained it."

The proportion of carers who were able to name a disease or illness in order to describe the older person's problems did not vary by social class. However, 80% of co-resident carers reported that they knew that the person for whom they cared had a diagnosis of Alzheimer's Disease or another type of dementia, compared with 56% of those living in a different household (χ^2=6.3, 1 df; p=0.01). Mrs Adams, who cared for her husband, commented.

"Alf has senile dementia. They call it Alzheimer's now, don't they?"

The proportion of co-resident carers who used a specific term to describe the older person's problems was higher than that reported in an earlier NISW study (Levin et al, 1994). However, at 65% the overall proportion of carers who reported that the person for whom they cared had Alzheimer's Disease or another form of dementia was only slightly higher. It represents a huge increase on the first NISW study, when just 5% of carers used one of these terms (E. Levin, personal communication), and is an indication of the greater public awareness of Alzheimer's Disease and other forms of dementia in recent years.

Most carers' understanding about what was the matter with the person for whom they cared had been obtained through consultations with health professionals, usually the GP or an old age psychiatrist. A minority, like Mrs Roberts, made a guess about what they felt was wrong. In some cases, they subsequently obtained confirmation from a professional. Six carers had found out through an accidental disclosure. For example one carer saw 'Alzheimer's Disease' written on a letter from her GP to the consultant old age psychiatrist. It was not clear whether the professionals involved in these cases had withheld information or whether they had assumed that the carer already knew.

The differing levels of knowledge among the carers is very consistent with the literature. One study found that the best informed carers were those attending an Alzheimer's Disease Society (ADS) support group (Graham et al, 1997). It suggested that community mental health teams and old age psychiatry services must regularly evaluate their methods of dissemination of knowledge to carers.

The second area in which carers identified a need for better information was in finding out what help was available to them and how to access it. Ms Lewis described her frustration in trying to find out who was the most appropriate agency to contact:

> *"Will she be like this for five or ten years or will she deteriorate next year? You are left trying to find these things out. I have spent hours on the 'phone. I don't know who I should turn to – never having been familiar with social services. [It] seems a great monolith – [I] don't know which door to bang on."*

In Chapter 4, we suggested that carers may now be better informed about how to access help from their local SSD than they were before the community care changes. However, considering that all the study participants had received an SSD assessment, it was disappointing that many carers seemed to be unaware of the full range of services that might be available. In particular, carers seemed to lack knowledge about home-based carer support, short-term care and the existence of carers' groups. This raises questions about the extent to which these carers were able to make informed choices about the most appropriate care solutions for themselves and for the person for whom they cared (Fisher, 1990b).

In addition to being unaware of what services were available, some carers were unfamiliar with the content of care plans and the levels of service delivery that had been agreed, particularly if they cared for someone living alone. Ms Lewis explained that she was not sure at what time the home care workers were supposed to visit her mother and what exactly they were meant to do while they were there. In a few cases communication between home care workers and non-resident carers was facilitated through link books, but these need to be regularly and clearly updated by service providers.

Voluntary organisations are another part of the network in which carers might find assistance. Carers were given a list of nine national organisations (Age Concern, Carers National

Association [CNA], Arthritis Care, Counsel and Care, RADAR, Parkinson's Disease Society, ADS, Care and Repair, and STROKE) and asked to state which ones they had heard of and whether they were a member of any (Moriarty and Webb, 1997). When the Time One data were being collected the Relatives' and Residents' Association had a lower national profile and so it was not included on the list. Carers had heard of an average of four (SD 2) organisations. Nearly everyone had heard of Age Concern. Three quarters knew about the ADS (whereas only half the carers in the respite care study had heard of it) (Levin et al, 1994). However, few carers were aware of Care and Repair (6%), Counsel and Care (18%) and CNA (31%). This is regrettable, as these three organisations could offer specific and very relevant assistance to people with dementia and their carers. Only 13% were members of any of the organisations named above. This suggests that there is potential for using assessments as a means of increasing carers' awareness of non-statutory sources of help.

Carers' social support and support from professionals

The identification of users' and carers' social networks and the practical and emotional support provided by friends and relatives is fundamental to the process of needs led assessment (Sheppard, 1995). There are two key reasons for this. First, the work of Wenger (1994b) suggests that networks focusing on local family ties may be more effective in maintaining people with dementia in the community than other network types. Second, social support may influence the psychological health of carers. It is not clear whether the presence of a confiding relationship acts as a buffer against stress, or whether it is the lack of a confiding relationship that is associated with poorer psychological health (Livingston et al, 1996).

We rated each carer's overall social support taking into account their contact with relatives and friends, the presence or absence of confiding relationships, and whether they had anyone who could undertake their caring role in the event of an emergency.

Four carers reported that they saw no friends or relatives regularly nor had anyone in whom they could confide or look to for help in an emergency; they were categorised as having no identified source of social support. Thirteen per cent had what was termed a single source; this meant that the carer relied on a single person for social contact, confidant and crisis support. Thirty-nine per cent had very limited social support; they did see friends or relatives occasionally and did have someone in whom they could confide, but there was no one with whom they could discuss everything. Forty-five per cent reported seeing a number of relatives or friends regularly and had several people in whom they confided; they were rated as having multiple support. Mr Williams, who cared for his mother-in-law, appreciated the benefits that this could bring:

"[I'm] lucky that [I] have a large close family that all live together."

Carers with none or limited support recognised their isolation. A few, such as Mr Theobald who cared for his wife, stated that this was through choice:

"There's only me ... I've finished with them [relatives].... I get on with my life and don't have to see them."

Wenger (1994b) has also described how social networks may become more restricted as a mental or physical health problem deteriorates. This was in line with the experience of Mrs Douglas, who had experienced a gradual withdrawing of support from friends as her husband's dementia became more apparent:

"It's three years since [my husband] was ill. Friends just eased off and then they never came at all, so it has been very lonely. [My neighbour] never came round to ask how [my husband] was or to ask if she could do any shopping for me. She came to the funeral and then came round twice to see if she could help, but what about the two and a half years before? She hasn't been round again."

Overall, only 30% of spouse carers had multiple sources of support, compared with 52% of other carers ($\chi^2=4.0$, 1 df; $p=0.04$).

Eighty-six per cent of carers could name at least one person (excluding professionals) in whom they were able to confide. Around half of them had

someone in whom they could confide most things. For spouse carers, their adult children were often the only or principal confidants mentioned. However, many spouse carers feel inhibited about discussing their caring situation with their children for fear of seeming disloyal to the parent with dementia. For non-spouse caregivers, partners and friends were important confidants. Some, like Mrs Nicholas caring for her mother, valued talking to others who had experience of caring:

"I can usually talk with my friend because she had a similar problem with her mother."

Despite the potential advantages to be gained from discussing caring experiences with others in a similar position, only 20% of the carers had ever attended a meeting of a carers' group. This compared with 28% of the carers who had participated in the respite care study (Levin et al, 1994). People who had attended carers' groups were usually positive about the experience, but Mrs Bryan, caring for her husband, had mixed feelings:

"Sharing troubles [is helpful] but [it] also frightens you hearing about future problems to be faced."

Just over a quarter of those who had never attended a carers' group would have liked the opportunity to attend.

Eleven per cent named a professional as one of the people to whom they could talk about problems, particularly those relating to caring. Eight carers mentioned their GP, two their social worker, and one person named both his social worker and the CPN. All but one of this group also had non-professional confidants. Other carers mentioned that they would ask professionals for advice, but not in the sense of confiding in anyone.

The evidence in Chapter 4 suggested that the highest levels of ongoing social work support were being focused on those who were finding caring most difficult. However, there were carers who wanted this kind of intervention and felt that they were missing out. Mrs Frederick had contacted her social worker but had received no response. She told the interviewer:

"I could have really done with help because I was scared."

Mrs Herbert explained that:

"Home care is fine, but I wish the social worker would contact me to find out how I am."

Supporting carers who cease to care

Although ceasing to care is associated with improvements in psychological health (Levin et al, 1989, 1994; Pushkar Gold et al, 1995), there is concern that some carers continue to experience difficulties in the short-term following their relatives' admission to long-term care. In particular, many carers feel guilty about reaching a decision to cease caring. When talking about his wife's move to a residential home, Mr Leonard said:

"I was critical of myself. I was disappointed that I hadn't improved enough to look after her. You can't wipe out 60 years of marriage, we're still very close."

Shortly after her sister's admission to a nursing home, Mrs Burt stated that:

"I worry a lot about [my sister].... I don't like to think of [her] in a nursing home. My other sister says I shouldn't worry because [my sister in the home] doesn't worry, but I can't help it."

Some carers who were currently caring were concerned about how they would manage in the event of becoming a former carer. A daughter explained:

"What happens when it [caring] stops?... Where does it leave the carer financially? There should be some short-term help while they get themselves sorted out because you lose various benefits, having saved the government thousands of pounds. I'm doing it because I want to and I don't want to see [my mother] in a home but I am concerned about the future for me – especially financially."

Discussion

Findings from the study suggested that, while there were many ways in which the carers' experiences reflected those to be found in earlier research, there were new influences as a result of demographic and social change.

Consistent with previous research, co-resident carers provided most care to the people with dementia in the study. They were less likely to receive help from other family members than non-resident carers, thus adding to the total amount of care for which they were responsible.

Although caring in itself may not be a risk factor for developing poor psychological health, a number of factors may contribute to carer stress. Assessments should be structured towards identifying which carers are especially likely to need assistance, and should not focus narrowly on the amount of personal care provided by the carer. Current carers found other aspects of caring – such as the presence of behavioural problems or the difficulty of maintaining social contacts – equally difficult.

A substantial proportion of former carers continued to provide direct assistance after the person for whom they cared had moved into long-term care. This suggested that residential and nursing homes in the study areas were increasingly working in partnership with those carers who wanted this degree of continuing involvement.

At the same time, there still needs to be better acknowledgement that carers may continue to experience difficulties, even after they have formally ceased to care. Some former carers had transport difficulties, which meant that they could not visit the person for whom they cared as often as they would have wished. In addition to providing help with hospital appointments or shopping trips, if volunteer transport, or local authority taxi-card and community transport schemes were also able to take visitors to residential and nursing homes, this would be a very worthwhile and useful form of assistance to former carers and would help to reduce the distress that many former carers feel.

Increased geographical mobility has meant that many non-resident carers have substantial journey times in order to visit the person for whom they care. It was notable that the carers who visited most often were those who lived within walking distance of the older person. In the long-term, new technology may offer the means of allowing carers and the people for whom they care to keep in contact. However, in the medium term there are likely to be increased demands on home care services to make more frequent visits to check on the safety of the person with dementia.

The proportion of carers in paid employment represents a shift from the earlier picture in which a disproportionate amount of caring was undertaken by women who were not in paid work. The government's strategy *Caring about carers* (Her Majesty's Government, 1999) has recognised the implications of this change and has offered support for the development of carer-friendly employment practices and support for carers to return to employment after a period of caregiving has ended. At the same time, we must recognise that it will take time before the effects of these changes are felt, and there must be help for the current generation of carers who are often in very difficult financial circumstances, as the proportion of carers with incomes of less than £10,000 per year showed.

Despite the number of studies and the work of organisations campaigning on behalf of carers that have pointed out the need to ensure that carers have access to information, we found that some carers had information needs that were not being met. In particular, carers need help from health services in improving their understanding of dementia, help from SSDs in realising what services are available, and access to other sources of help from national and local voluntary organisations.

At the same time, it should be recognised that carers of people with dementia may benefit from ongoing social work support. Spouse carers provided higher levels of help and supervision which may have led to poorer psychological ill-health. They appeared to have lower overall levels of social support, and many lacked a confidant with whom they felt able to discuss the strains and stresses of caring. It is essential that the work of CPNs and social workers continues to recognise the importance of providing support to carers who may have no other means of sharing their anxieties and difficulties.

Having considered the provision of information and support in this chapter, the next one looks at practical assistance in the form of the provision of community services to the older people and their carers.

Service packages

Key points

- This chapter focuses on services provided to study participants living in the community at Time One.

- The majority received at least one of the following: home care, day care, meals, home-based carer support, and short-term care. Home care and day care were used most frequently.

- Overall community-based service packages were not intensive, but there was evidence that home care was being tailored to meet the special needs of people with dementia.

- The use of services designed to meet carers' needs for a break, such as short-term care or home-based carer support, was limited.

- The overall pattern of service receipt did not change markedly between Time One and Time Two for people who continued to live at home.

- Case examples show how services were combined into packages and illustrate the range of views that the older people and carers expressed about the services that they received.

"We didn't realise how much help is available; we got more help than I thought we would." (Mrs Roy, caring for her non-resident mother-in-law)

Introduction

In Chapter 3, we explained that by Time One, approximately six months after their referral, around two thirds (*n*=84) of the 132 people residing in the community when they were referred were still living at home. In this chapter we look at the services that members of this group received. The analyses exclude the four people with dementia with no proxy informant or carer, because verification of whether a service was used or not was provided by proxy informants and carers. In their case, there was no one with whom we could confirm precise details of service receipt.

Previous research has shown that people with dementia tend to be multiple service users, and that the overall number of services they receive tends be greater than that received by other groups of older people (O'Connor et al, 1989a; Livingston et al, 1990; Philp et al, 1995; Burholt et al, 1997). Over time, their service use tends to increase (Cullen et al, 1993).

With some exceptions (Challis et al, 1997; Livingston et al, 1997), studies of cross-service use by people with dementia have generally reported which services were used and the total number of services received. Such approaches have their limitations. For instance, in analyses based simply on the numbers of services received, a person with 15 hours of home care per week might appear to be receiving less support than someone with an hour's home care and meals-on-wheels five days a week.

The first NISW dementia study (Levin et al, 1989) suggested that the key to success in maintaining older people with dementia at home lay in the *overall* package, rather than *individual* service receipt. The second (Levin et al, 1994) found some links between the numbers of respite services used and the severity of dementia. However, it also pointed out how variation in provision between different parts of the country could influence what services were received. Thus, people receiving day care and short-term care were very similar to those receiving day care, short-term care and home-based carer support. The difference between these two groups was not that they had different needs but that, where day care and short-term care only were being used, there was very limited provision of home-based carer support. In the study area where people used all three services, the limited amount of day care provision meant that, overall, those receiving all three respite services did not have more service than those with two.

The evidence outlined above suggested that a more comprehensive approach than considering individual service receipt was required. This is why this chapter gives examples of service combinations, reports on how often and for how long services were provided each week, and describes changes to service use between Times One and Two.

Services for people living in the community at Time One

Almost all the people with dementia living at home at Time One (which took place during the financial year 1995/96) received at least one community care service, defined as home care, day care, a home-based carer support service, a meals service or short-term care. Table 6.1 shows how few people living at home at Time One received none of these services. All eight had carers, although four lived alone. In most cases, either the person with dementia or his or her carer had refused services. Mrs Benjamin, living alone in metropolitan borough, explained:

"I do everything myself and never ask anybody. I don't need it."

In Chapter 4 we mentioned that assessing and arranging services in a way that respected the preferences of people with dementia required sensitivity on the part of assessors and carers. Mr Gilbert who cared for his mother told the interviewer:

"[Services are] not necessary at the moment and mother wouldn't like it. They are leaving it to me, if it gets too much for me, to contact them."

As Table 6.1 shows, the main services provided were home care and day care; 29% of the people with dementia had received at least one short-term break in the three years before the Time One interview; 18% had a meals service, usually meals-on-wheels. In view of the increasing emphasis on meeting carers' needs since the community care changes, it was striking how unusual it was for people to receive a home-based carer support service.

Table 6.1: Receipt of community care services at Time One

	n	%
Home care	48	60
Day care	46	58
Short-term care	23	29
Meals service	14	18
Home-based carer support	7	9
None of the above	8	10
Base *n*	80	100

Apart from some day care and day hospital provision, most services were provided generically and were not specifically aimed at people with dementia. About three quarters of people with home care had local authority home care workers, and the remainder had workers who were employed by private agencies. We made a distinction between home care, where the emphasis was on assistance with personal care, shopping and meal preparation, and home-based carer support, where it was on providing the people with dementia with an opportunity for social interaction and where the visit lasted long enough to enable the carer to have a break from caring. While this type of service is nationally mainly provided by Crossroads or the

Alzheimer's Society, in this study it was almost always purchased from private agencies. Day care attendance was almost equally distributed between the NHS, local authority and voluntary organisation providers.

The only services for which there were sufficient users to compare provision between the study areas were home care, day care and short-term care. The provision of home care and short-term care did not differ significantly between the study areas, but almost three quarters of the people with dementia living in the county council received day care compared with half of those living in the London or metropolitan boroughs (χ^2=4.9; 1 df; p=0.03). Fewer people in the metropolitan borough received both home care and day care.

Charging for community care services

We collected details at Times One and Two of the charges that study participants paid for community care services and have reported on this elsewhere (Moriarty and Webb, 1998).

While there is a national system for means testing the charges for residential and nursing home care, each authority has its own system for setting charges for community care services. Most local authorities have undertaken major reviews of their charging policies in the years following the implementation of the 1990 National Health Service and Community Care Act. In general, there has been a shift from flat charges for community services towards means testing. At the time the data were collected during the financial years 1995/96 and 1996/97, each authority had set a maximum charge that could be levied. All three were committed to keeping charges for non-residential community care services as low as possible. Day care and meals services seemed to be charged at flat rates. Home care and short-term care charges appeared to be levied in bands relating to the older person's income and the period of service receipt. Day hospital care was free at the point of delivery, as was short-term care in NHS venues. Two thirds of the older people living at home at Time One appeared to have an annual income of less than £10,000. This has implications for the proportion of the costs of care

that would be recouped from this group, and from other older people in similar financial circumstances. The Audit Commission has drawn attention to the wide variation in current charging policies and has identified a need to set clear objectives and targets in charging (Audit Commission, 1999).

Numbers and types of services received

The mean number of services received was two (SD 1), with 31% (n=22) of the people using community care services receiving two services and 29% (n=21) receiving three or more. Only one person received the maximum of five community-based services. The *number* of services received was not associated with living alone, with the type of carer (spouse, daughter, other) or with the severity of dementia. However, consistent with previous studies (Levin et al, 1989; 1994; O'Connor et al, 1989a; Philp et al, 1995), there were associations between the characteristics of the people with dementia and their carers according to the *types* of services received.

Where service receipt consisted of home care or a combination of home care and meals, study participants were more likely to live alone.

Case example

Mrs James lived alone and was visited by her nephew, Mr Richards, twice a week. The only service she received was home care. Mrs James' severe dementia (she scored 8 on the OBS) meant that she was unable to offer an opinion on the service when interviewed. However, Mr Richards explained: "She's not very complimentary at times. She feels her independence is threatened. [From my point of view], the main thing is that someone calls in daily so I know she'll be OK." At Time One, this was her care plan:

Day	Home care
Monday	9.30 to 10.30
Tuesday	9.30 to 10.30
Wednesday	9.30 to 10.30
Thursday	9.30 to 10.30
Friday	9.30 to 10.30
Saturday	Pop in for one hour – no specified time
Sunday	Pop in for one hour – no specified time

Table 6.2: Receipt of home care and meals services by type of carer and severity of dementia

	Receives either home care or meals or both		Valid *n*	Significance (1 df)
	Yes	No		
Type of carer				$\chi^2=12.36; p=0.001$
% with co-resident carer	40	60	30	
% with non-resident carer	80	20	41	
% sample with carers (*n*)	63 (45)	37 (26)	71	
Severity of dementia				NS
% mild to moderate (OBS=3-7)	68	32	47	
% severe (OBS=8)	65	35	20	
% sample (*n*)	67 (45)	33 (22)	67	

This example is reflected in the data presented in Table 6.2, which shows that people with non-resident carers were more likely to receive home care or a combination of home care and meals. It also shows that severity of dementia was not associated with receipt of these services.

Consistent with the existing literature (O'Connor et al, 1989a; Levin et al, 1989; 1994), combinations that included day care, home-based carer support or short-term care were used especially by people with co-resident carers and with more severe dementia.

In addition to the association between type of service receipt and type of carer, Table 6.3 also shows that people with severe dementia were more likely to use day care only or a combination of day care and short-term care.

People receiving both home care and day care were more likely to be cared for by daughters. This probably reflects daughters' greater willingness to seek and accept sources of outside help in comparison with spouse carers (Twigg et al, 1990).

Case example

Mrs Douglas cared for her husband, "out of duty and affection", but found it "wearing looking after him." Mr Douglas had very severe dementia. He was incontinent and was no longer able to speak. Their only son lived abroad and they saw no friends or relatives regularly. "It's all to do with [my husband's condition]. Otherwise I'd see people more and do things." Mr Douglas received both day care and short-term care, help that Mrs Douglas appreciated. "I've just got to have the help and be thankful for what help I do get. At the moment I don't think I want anything else."

Day	Day care	Regular short-term care
Monday	None	Six weeks at home, two weeks in local authority home
Tuesday	10.00 to 15.30	
Wednesday	None	
Thursday	10.00 to 15.30	
Friday	None	
Saturday	None	
Sunday	10.00 to 15.30	

Table 6.3: Receipt of day care, home-based carer support, and short-term care by type of carer and severity of dementia

| | Receives day care or home-based carer support and/ or short-term care | | Valid *n* | Significance (1 df) |
	Yes	No		
Type of carer				$\chi^2=6.8; p=0.008$
% with co-resident carer	83	17	30	
% with non-resident carer	54	46	41	
% sample with carer (*n*)	66 (47)	34 (24)	71	
Severity of dementia				$\chi^2=4.7; p=0.03$
% mild to moderate (OBS=3-7)	43	57	47	
% severe (OBS=8)	85	15	20	
% sample (*n*)	66 (44)	34 (23)	67	

Case example

Mrs Owen lived alone and was cared for by her son-in-law and daughter, Mr and Mrs Michaels.

Day	Home care	Day care
Monday	8.30 to 9.30	9.30 to 15.30
Tuesday	10.00 to 11.00	None
Wednesday	None	10.00 to 15.00
Thursday	10.00 to 11.00	None
Friday	10.00 to 11.00	None
Saturday	None	None
Sunday	None	None

Mrs Owen had severe dementia (her OBS score was 8). The home care worker helped her get up, wash and dress. Then she made her breakfast. Mrs Owen described her as 'lovely'. Mr Michaels confirmed this, "On her good days, she gives [home care worker] glowing comments." Mrs Owen spent Mondays and Wednesdays at two different local day centres. On the days when she did not attend day care, she went to Mr and Mrs Michaels' house for her main meal; afterwards, they took her home. Mr and Michaels also visited her on Monday and Wednesday evenings. They were pleased with her care plan as it meant that they did not have to help her get up in the mornings and day care gave them 'days off'. Mr Michaels said, "From our limited experience it seems to work really well. At present, we're coping all right."

In this section we have looked at examples of the overall package of services provided to the study participants. The next part of the chapter reports on the frequency, intensity and content of each service and presents the views of the carers and of the older people who used the services.

Home care

"It's keeping her healthy and safe in her own home and still giving her the independence she wants." (Mrs Franks, caring for her non-resident mother)

Home care was provided an average of seven times per week (SD 5), spread over five days (SD 2). The average length of visit was 45 minutes (SD 22). Within this, there was a great deal of variation. The shortest visit lasted five minutes, the longest an hour and a half. The minimum visit per week was one; the maximum was 21. In total, home care users received an average of five hours' (SD 3) help per week. The minimum amount of home care provided per week was 45 minutes and the maximum was 14 hours.

Although nearly every carer and proxy informant knew how long each home care visit was supposed to last, a third (*n*=15) could not give a precise timing for the visits. Sometimes this was because they did not know. Others reported that the workers did not arrive at a regular time.

Most visits took place between 7.00 and 10.00 am, in order to help the older person get up. The home care workers also undertook other tasks, including help with cooking (discussed more fully in the section on meals), as well as the more traditional housework and shopping. A positive finding was that 44% of home care users received the service over the weekend, although far fewer (*n*=7) received a visit after 5.00 pm.

One of the most important issues identified in research completed prior to April 1993 was the comparative lack of support given to co-resident carers of people with dementia by traditional home help services (O'Connor et al, 1989a; Levin et al, 1989). This caused concern because of the overwhelming evidence that those receiving the least help from traditional home care services were co-resident carers of people with the most severe dementia.

In an earlier NISW study (Levin et al, 1994), co-resident carers assisted the people for whom they cared in an average of six ADLs (SD 3), yet the average ADL assistance from services totalled less than one (0.8, SD 1). This generally consisted of help leaving the house in order to attend day care. In this study, co-resident carers assisted with five ADLs (SD 3) and services assisted with 2 ADLs (SD 2).

Taken as a whole, our findings on the content and timing of home care visits would appear to reflect the wider trend towards providing a more intensive home care service, albeit to fewer people. The data set from this study is not strictly comparable with the earlier NISW research (Levin et al, 1994). However, in the absence of studies that were actually designed to compare community-based services before and after April 1993, it may be taken as giving some support to the impression that changes to home care services have resulted in some improved support to co-resident carers of people with dementia.

Almost all the carers believed that both they and the people for whom they cared benefited from the service. Non-resident carers, like Mrs Scott who cared for her cousin, valued regular home care visits for the reassurance it gave them that someone was checking on the older person's physical well being:

"I feel that someone is looking after my cousin now. It has helped knowing that someone is going in to see she is okay."

They also valued the social aspects of the visit for the older person. Mr Barnaby who cared for his mother said:

"Human contact is important."

In common with their carers, many of the people with dementia appreciated the practical help provided by home care. Miss Dennis, living alone in the county council district, described what the home care worker did:

"She bustles around a bit and we have a talk and a cup of tea.... People like that can be very helpful, nice to give me a rest."

Many of the older people who lived alone, like Mrs Kenny, also valued the social aspect:

"It's somebody to talk to. They're the only ones I see."

Day care

"It's taken a lot of pressure off us. If my mother-in-law had not gone to day care, I would have had to give up work, which I don't want to do. It's my release from looking after her. (Mrs Roy, caring for her non-resident mother-in-law)

People attending day care at Time One received an average of 19 hours day care (SD 13) spread over three days a week (SD 3). Once more, there was wide variation in service receipt, ranging from someone who had just one day's care that lasted four and a half hours to another who attended seven days a week for nine hours per day. In contrast to home care, where it was not unusual to receive the service at the weekend, only six people attended day care on either Saturday or Sunday.

Just over half of the carers rated day care as making their life better and another 42% said that it was much better. As with home care, carers such as Mrs Franks often emphasised its social benefits:

"It means she gets other company. I can't be all to her, she needs more than me."

Some people with dementia did indeed enjoy the company provided by day care. Mrs George who lived alone in the London borough told the interviewer:

"I go on a Monday. We yap and eat. It's surprising how time passes. When you've been going for a bit you get used to it. It's friendly."

Others enjoyed a change from being at home, but a few, such as Mrs Lewis, found it an ordeal:

"It seemed a long time and I was glad to get home. My memory is not as good as it was and I would rather not go than say the wrong thing or upset someone."

Short-term care

"My aunt enjoyed the company, the food and the surroundings.... It made a big difference. We had a worry-free holiday." (Mr Lester, caring for his aunt, Mrs Graham)

"We all get together and have a sing song or a walk in the grounds. It was comfortable but not like home." (Mrs Graham, living alone in the metropolitan borough)

Researching short-term care poses methodological problems not encountered in services that are received on a daily or weekly basis. Intervals between breaks might vary from four to 52 weeks, making it difficult to distinguish between regular and occasional use. Long intervals between breaks can result in respondents having problems with recall.

Twenty-nine per cent of the people with dementia living in the community at Time One had received one or more short-term breaks. Two others had used the service once but not within the last three years. In the interval between the two interviews, a third of those living at home at Time One went on to receive short-term care. Six people did not use the service again because they went into long-term care or died. Time Two users were almost equally divided between 'new' users (those for whom the service had started since Time One) and 'continuous' users (those who received breaks throughout the study period). With one exception, short-term care was used in conjunction with another regular community service, most frequently day care and/or home care.

Two thirds of the 30 people with co-resident carers used short-term care at least once during the study period in comparison with a third of the people with dementia with a non-resident carer or no carer (χ^2=9.8; 2 df; p=0.002). Three quarters of the people with co-resident carers who received short-term care went to NHS hospital wards or local authority homes, showing that these settings continue to comprise the dominant form of short-stay provision.

There has been a longstanding debate about whether short-term care precipitates or delays entry into long-term care. In Chapter 7 we shall show that receipt of short-term care was not associated with entry to long-term care in this study. Four people with co-resident carers moved into long-term care immediately following a short-term stay. Two people were admitted to short-term care following an illness of their carer that ultimately proved to be too severe to enable the older person to return home. Two older people were intended to receive regular breaks but their carers felt unable to continue and so they were admitted to residential care. By contrast, seven of the nine people without a co-resident carer either did not return home from their stay or were admitted to long-term care within days of their return home. The other two received the service as an emergency.

Unlike day care and home care, where carers were likely to see the service as equally beneficial for them and the person for whom they cared, short-term care aroused more ambivalent feelings. While most carers valued having time off from caring, they were more likely to see it as being of mixed benefit to the older person. This was why finding the right venue could play a part in deciding whether or not to have the service. Mrs Timothy, caring for her husband, explained to the interviewer why she had given up the service:

"The first time was good. It was a little home and he was treated as part of the family. He settled quickly and enjoyed himself. They seemed to know how to treat him. But they stopped doing short-term breaks so the only place he could go was All Saints Hospital. I'd love a chance to catch up with friends, but not if it means him going to All Saints."

Meals services

"Not too good! Get a lot of mashed potatoes." (Mrs Williams, cared for by her husband and daughter)

Eighteen per cent (*n*=14) of people living at home at Time One received a meals service. With two exceptions, meals were provided in conjunction with home care. Apart from one older person who attended a lunch club and another who went to a local café for lunch, meals were delivered by local authority or voluntary sector meals-on-wheels.

Traditional meals services have been criticised for not providing appropriate support for people with dementia living at home (O'Connor et al, 1989a). However, carers and proxy informants reported that half of the people receiving home care were given help with meal preparation by home care staff. When these figures are combined, the proportion of people who received help with meals rose to 36% of all those living at home. Half of those living alone received help with meal preparation or meals-on-wheels compared with 17% of those living with one or more others (χ^2= 9.8, 1 df; *p*=0.002).

Assistance with meal preparation was generally appreciated by carers. One daughter, caring for her mother who lived alone, said:

"It cuts down on the things I have to do. I know she gets lunch and [otherwise] I couldn't have worked. It would have been impossible."

Traditional meals-on-wheels services received more criticism. It included complaints about the lack of choice, the quality and presentation of the food, and the timing of meal deliveries. This was less likely to occur when food was prepared in the older person's home using ingredients that took account of the older person's dietary preferences. It also reduced

the likelihood that a person with dementia might forget to eat the meal, as sometimes happens with a simple delivery service.

Home-based carer support

"It was wonderful! I could have a good night's sleep." (Mrs Barry, caring for her husband)

Carers and proxy informants were asked what the home care workers did during their visits. From their replies, it appeared that home care workers made a point of chatting to around 40% of the people with dementia using the service. However, this was incidental to providing assistance with meals or personal care, suggesting that providing the older person with social activities and stimulation did not appear to be a core feature of the home care service.

Overall, only seven people (representing less than a third of the 30 people with a co-resident carer) had a home-based care service designed to enable the carer to go out and to provide social activities for the older person. This proportion is very low, even allowing for the traditional focus of these schemes on supporting co-resident carers who formed a minority in our sample. No one received an intensive service, with carers typically receiving a few hours each week purchased from the local authority home care service or a private agency. Only one person received overnight care.

In contrast to meals where assistance from home care reflected a positive change from traditional forms of service delivery, the failure to provide home-based care tailored to the special needs of people with dementia meant that the only way in which study participants could be encouraged to retain social skills and maintain hobbies and interests was through attending day care.

The few carers who did use home-based carer support appreciated the brief respite it gave. All would have liked more. Mrs Harold, caring for her husband, had a home-based carer support worker for three and a half hours every Wednesday afternoon to allow her to go to an art class. She said:

63

"[It's] essential to get out when I can. I really need to keep going to my class."

Mr Harold obviously enjoyed the sitter's visits:

"We just chat together, television maybe. She's a very satisfactory person."

As we mentioned in Chapter 5, few carers were familiar with this form of care, suggesting that it may not be routinely discussed when care plans are being arranged. This is disappointing, as previous research has indicated that many carers favour the idea of home-based carer support and would be willing to try the service were it to be available (Levin et al, 1994). Mrs Ivor would have liked the 'brain relief' that home-based carer support would offer from caring for her husband. Mr Noel would have valued being able to:

"... go out and know she's [wife] all right. She's not safe with electrical appliances."

Comments from the people with dementia showed that some of them were also aware of the opportunities that such a service might bring them.

Case example

Mrs Luke had been widowed for many years. She had no children. Her niece and her niece's husband lived some distance away, although they visited when they could. A home care worker visited three times a day, seven days a week and Mrs Luke also had meals-on-wheels. She had mild to moderate dementia, scoring 4 on the OBS. Her regular home care worker had been ill. Mrs Luke found the changes difficult to deal with. "I have so many people. Two or three people come in, it's a job to remember.... It's a long time from lunch or tea-time right through to the next morning.... Nobody comes in and says 'We're going for a walk.' I've got a nice pram [?reference to wheelchair].... I would like them to take me out.... I don't feel unhappy [but I do feel lonely] sometimes. Not terribly lonely. I just sit here and watch."

Health services

Sixty-nine per cent of those living in the community had seen their GP in the three months before Time One, a higher proportion than that reported in the GHS, which contains data on service use among a nationally representative sample of people living in private households (Bennett et al, 1996); 24% of study participants were reported to have seen a district nurse and 15% a CPN. As Chapter 8 shows, most contact with community nurses centred primarily on assessment visits and did not comprise part of the weekly package of care. Fifty-six per cent were reported to have seen an old age psychiatrist. This is a higher proportion than in two community samples of people with dementia (Burholt et al, 1997). The most probable explanation for the difference is sample selection. Our sample sources included eight specialist teams where a high proportion of clients are likely to have been seen by a consultant psychiatrist (Coles et al, 1991). Just under a half of the older people had been to the optician; a fifth had seen a dentist; 60% had seen a chiropodist.

Privately arranged services

Only 11 people with dementia used any services that had been arranged without assistance from the SSD. Eight people paid for help with cleaning. Four people had a gardener. Only three people paid for personal care. (These numbers include four people who used two privately arranged services.) Although we did not systematically record whether dental and chiropody services had been arranged privately or on the NHS, it appeared from some of the carers' comments that these services were purchased privately more frequently than housework or social care services.

Service use between Time One and Time Two

The overall pattern of service receipt for those in the community did not change substantially between Times One and Two. Home care and day care continued to be the main services provided. Consistent with the literature, most service users at Time One continued to be service users if they had remained living at home (Cullen et al, 1993). The most frequent change to care plans involved the cessation of all community-based services upon the older person's entry into long-term care or upon his or her death. For example, Mrs James, who had received home care for an hour every day, had the same level of service until her entry into a residential home.

The majority of those still living in the community at Time Two (*n*=44) had experienced at least one change to their care plan. Just over half had had a change to the type of service they received since Time One, with the most frequent new service being short-term care. Some changes were made following reviews or other contact from social services. For example, Mr and Mrs Douglas received a visit from a new social worker who supplemented his existing care package by arranging for home care visits to help Mr Douglas get up in the morning and into bed at night. Mrs Douglas stopped the service after a few months:

> *"In some ways it was a waste of time. They came at 7.30 am and dressed him, but then he wet everything and I had to dress him again before the day centre."*

Shortly afterwards, Mr Douglas collapsed and was admitted to hospital where he died.

Almost half of those who remained at home had some change to the amount of services they received.

Case example

At Time Two Mrs Owen was still living alone in the community. No changes had been made to the types of service that she received but there had been other adjustments to the care package. The social worker had suggested that Mrs Owen attend day care on a third day. This meant that she was now spending less time on her own. In an example of good service coordination, the timing of Mrs Owen's Friday home care visit had been altered so that the workers came earlier on Fridays to help her get up in time for day care.

Day	Home care	Day care
Monday	8.30 to 9.30	9.30 to 15.00
Tuesday	10.00 to 11.00	None
Wednesday	None	10.00 to 15.00
Thursday	10.00 to 11.00	None
Friday	8.30 to 9.00	9.30 to 15.00
Saturday	None	None
Sunday	None	None

Her covers, Mr and Mrs Michaels, said that they would consider long-term care only if Mrs Owen's condition deteriorated.

Some changes had been made subsequent to hospital admission and discharge. A few carers contacted the SSD themselves to request a service. In six cases there was an overall reduction in service receipt.

Case example

Mr Craig, who cared for his mother who lived alone, reported that they had seen neither the assessor nor anyone else from the SSD between Times One and Two. At Time One, Mrs Craig had attended day care, but she changed her mind and refused to go anymore. Mr Craig was not sure why this had happened. "I've not the faintest idea.... She liked it at first and then she just said she wasn't going again." No alternatives had been offered although Mr Craig would have liked both home care and day care. "[Day care] would give me a free day where I'd be able to do my shopping or whatever. [Home care] would make sure she got her tablets and had food if I was ill and couldn't get round." His own health was poor and he was concerned about his mother's future care. "If I got worse, I suppose it wouldn't be long before we would have to get help or something."

Discussion

The finding that home care and day care were the main community services provided reflects earlier work and shows the continuing importance of these services in the support of older people with dementia and their carers in the community (SSI, 1997).

The most important factor influencing use of home care was household size, with this service being used most often by those living alone. However, 40% of co-resident carers had assistance from home care, meaning that the people with dementia were not entirely reliant upon their carers for help with personal care. The use of workers from one agency to assist people to get ready to attend day care provided by another organisation raises questions about whether there is potential for better co-ordination. What happens if the home care workers arrive late and the transport to day care is early? Alternatively, as many carers will testify, a long gap between getting up and actually leaving the house for day care can be very stressful for some people with dementia. One possibility would be for pilot schemes in which day care providers are assisted in

developing a linked home care service in which clients could be helped to get ready in the morning and then accompanied to day care.

The carers' comments suggested that, when home care workers provided help with meal preparation, this was a more appropriate response to the needs of people with dementia. This is one example where changes to the traditional home help and meals-on-wheels services appear to have resulted in services that are more suited to the needs of carers and people with dementia.

One of the concerns expressed by those supporting a rights-based, rather than a needs-based, approach to community care is the way in which social participation appears to be viewed simply as 'occasional add-on' to personal care (Lindow, 1999). This was certainly reflected in the finding that, apart from assistance with personal care or meal preparation, few other forms of home-based care were provided. It is disappointing partly because the community care changes were aimed at encouraging the development of more flexible and creative packages of care, and partly because there is evidence that an augmented domiciliary service (Riordan and Bennett, 1998), or intensive home care provision as part of a specialist care management service (Challis et al, 1997), can help people with dementia to remain at home. The reliance upon day care as the prime way of meeting a person with dementia's needs for leisure and social contact means that people with dementia are at risk of social exclusion if they do not wish to attend day care, or if their mobility or psychological care needs are too great to be met in day centres with a standard ratio of staff to clients.

The apparent difference in the levels of provision of day care between the study areas, with people in the metropolitan borough being less likely to receive the service, is of particular concern in view of the fact that, as in previous research (Levin et al, 1989; 1994), day care continues to be one of the main ways in which people with dementia are supported in the community. It was the main service offering carers a regular break.

Short-term care had generally been added to existing services to take account of increased needs for care among the people with dementia or increased levels of stress in the carer (Levin et al, 1994). The variation in the intensity of short-term care and in the purposes for which it is provided supports calls for greater specificity in defining what constitutes this type of care. Analyses of the effectiveness of short-term care must be able to control for potentially confounding factors (such as the greater severity of dementia among its users or increased levels of stress among their carers) which might lead to the false assumption that the service accelerates entry to long-term care. Without this, it will remain difficult to evaluate service effectiveness properly (Brodaty and Gresham, 1992; Nolan and Grant, 1992; Moriarty and Levin, 1998).

Comments from the carers and people with dementia show the need to increase the range of mainstream community services. Home-based services provided reassurance for non-resident carers and offered practical support with ADLs and IADLs. However, efforts should be made to expand the focus of these services so that they can also cater for the social and leisure needs of people with dementia and support for their carers. Short-term care continued to be provided mainly in residential homes and hospitals. The implication of this will be discussed more fully in Chapter 8. Unless it is being provided because the person with dementia has health care needs that require treatment, hospital-based respite care is extremely expensive in comparison to other forms of short stay care. The actual venue for respite care can be instrumental in governing whether or not the stay is successful, as the comments from carers and people with dementia showed. The development of overnight home-based care or helping providers of small residential homes to expand into short-term care should be encouraged.

The data on what services were received and for how long show that, overall, community-based service packages were not intensive. This will be explained further in Chapter 8, which costs the packages of care received by study participants.

However, most of those who remained living in the community at Time Two had experienced changes either to the types of service they received or to the frequency and intensity of existing services. In some cases adjustments were made following formal reviews, but in others changes were independent of

the care management process. The nature of dementia is such that reviews are unlikely to result in reductions to the package of care that is required. However, it is essential that such reviews do take place because, over time, the need for care among people with dementia will increase. They also provide the opportunity for discussing whether alternative forms of help are available in instances where the carer or person with dementia has stopped a particular service.

In the next chapter we shall consider whether community services played a part in enabling participants to remain in their own homes as we return to examine what happened to all 141 study participants.

7

Care paths

Key points

- This chapter discusses factors influencing whether study participants remained at home or entered long-term care.

- Over an 18-month period, around 60% of those living in the community at referral went into long-term care.

- While severity of dementia was the strongest predictor of entry into long-term care, other factors included whether or not the person had a carer and the receipt of home care and day care.

- Behavioural problems appeared to have greatest impact on current co-resident carers.

- Helping people with dementia adjust to living in long-term care is a very important role for staff working in long-term care.

- The proportion of people with depression in long-term care is a cause for concern.

- Former carers seemed to find that the transition from caring for someone living at home was easier with time.

- There were examples of good practice in supporting former carers who wished to remain involved in the care of the person with dementia.

"It's difficult to answer [what would be best for families]. I'd say keep the [person with dementia] at home for as long as they could. Get access to services and consider residential care when it becomes too much. The trouble is getting the right package of care." (Ms Lindsay, home manager and proxy informant)

"I accepted home care [because] I was too ill to do anything. Eric [husband] loved day care and it was a big help to me [but] he became too difficult to look after.... He liked it at Green Lodge [short stay venue].... The stays were planned for two weeks every other fortnight.... I felt guilty but it did give me a break.... When he came home he wanted to go back [to Green Lodge] because he missed it. That made me feel dreadful, terrible. I was suicidal. When Eric went to Green Lodge [for short stays] I was told not to see him and that made me feel bad too, guilty.... For me, [short stays] made me a bit better physically but when he came back I was back where I started.... He was moved to Woodland View [nursing home].... I just couldn't cope any more. I don't want Eric [to be] in Woodland View but I can't look after him." (Mrs Duncan, interviewed at Time Two)

"I want to go home, or somewhere where I can look after myself but there's nothing wrong with being here.... I'd just like to be somewhere where I can look after myself but they're very kind here." (Mrs Dominic, one year after admission into long-term care)

Introduction

The opening quotations set the theme for this chapter, which emphasises that what happened to participants over the study period was the result of a series of complex and interrelated factors. It draws together some of the themes from earlier chapters and sets the context for the following chapter which discusses the costs of packages of care.

The circumstances of referrals to the study SSDs highlighted the long-term nature of the model of service delivery that would be required. The overwhelming majority of assessments had resulted in service changes, and response times and the steps taken to involve carers in assessments reflected positively on the performance of the SSDs at the time of the study. While it is more difficult to demonstrate effective performance in terms of practice skills, this is not, in itself, a justification for ignoring the issue. While all the carers interviewed in the study provided substantial levels of support in terms of practical help and contact, it was current co-resident carers who gave most assistance. They generally had less help from other members of their family and friends and lower levels of social support. There were some signs that community care services had become more responsive to the needs of people with dementia and their carers in terms of providing more intensive assistance and offering help with personal care and meal preparation. However, short-term care and day care were still being provided in very traditional ways. As Chapter 8 will show, the costs of community services were similar to those in residential care.

At the time of referral, almost all the study participants lived in the community. By Time Two, on average some 18 months later, the proportion was less than a third. Why should some study participants have remained at home while others went into long-term care? The study design enabled us to look at this question closely.

The role of assessment in determining admission to long-term care

The highest costs of social work time in assessments occur where health services are involved, where there is carer or family involvement, where more than one sector is involved in the provision of care, and where long-term care is required (Levin et al, 1997). Chapter 4 showed that there was substantial involvement from carers and health professionals in assessments. Chapter 6 explained that a number of people received a combination of community care services. Furthermore, although SSD assessments can be completed by qualified or unqualified staff, it was notable that nearly all the study participants had been assessed by a qualified social worker, which is another factor contributing to social work costs. By implication, the costs of assessing study participants in terms of social work time are likely to have been considerable.

However, the costs of social work time in assessment can be offset by the sustainability of the care packages they arrange. Data from the five month interval between assessment and the Time One interviews suggested that the assessors had made successful judgements about whether or not continued residence in the community was feasible. Almost 60% of the assessments (*n*=81) had resulted in an offer of one or more of the following services: home care, other home-based carer support, day care, meals or short-stay care. Just over a quarter had resulted in an offer of residential or nursing care, reflecting the way in which many referrals to SSDs take place when the risk of entry into long-term care is already high. In the interval between the assessment and Time One, another 20 people went into long-term care. Of these, seven were examples of self-funding people where the admission had been arranged by the family without further reference to the assessor. In one instance, it was a change in the older person's physical health that had precipitated the admission; in another, carer illness had meant that the person with dementia had to go into long-term care. Two people with dementia had refused the services offered at assessment but crises had occurred and they were then admitted to long-term care. Overall, this gives support to the viewpoint that the assessors were not setting up large numbers of community-based packages of care which quickly broke down.

Comparisons between people living in the community and those in long-term care

One of the chief reasons behind the community care changes was a concern that people were moving into long-term care when their needs could have been met by a lower level of service receipt. The theme of promoting independence continues to be one of the main principles underpinning

Modernising social services (Secretary of State for Health, 1998), as is shown by the requirement that health authorities and SSDs draw up joint investment plans for avoiding unnecessary hospital or care home admissions.

Table 7.1 uses scores on the OBS and DEP scales from the BAS (Macdonald et al, 1982) to compare people living in long-term care at Time One with those living in the community. It shows that proportionally more people in long-term care had severe dementia and had depression. Overall, the mean scores of people in long-term care on both the OBS and the DEP were higher.

Table 7.1: BAS OBS (Dementia) and DEP (Depression) scale scores*

	% all	% in the community	% in any long-term care
Dementia			
Mild to moderate (OBS=3-7)	64	70	53
Severe (OBS=8)	36	30	47
Base *n*	118	71	47
Depression			
Depressed (DEP=7-24)	29	21	45
Not depressed (DEP=0-6)	71	79	55
Base *n*	82	53	29
***Dementia**			
Mean OBS scores			*p*=0.0004
People in the community		5.9 (SD 1.8)	(*n*=71)
People in long-term care		7.0 (SD 1.2)	(*n*=47)
Depression			
Mean DEP scores			*p*=0.052
People in the community		4.1 (SD 3.7)	(*n*=53)
People in long-term care		5.9 (SD 4.3)	(*n*=29)

Table 7.2: Help with ADLs and IADLs from services and from carers

	Mean rank			
	Community	Long-term care	U	Significance of U
Help from services				
N ADLs where services help	40.90	91.13	378.0	0.0000
N IADLs where services help	37.88	84.15	317.5	0.0000
Base *n*	70	55		
Help from carers				
N ADLs where carer helps	59.27	29.36	411.5	0.0000
N IADLs where carer helps	58.70	18.41	119.0	0.0000
Base *n*	66	27		

Table 7.2 looks at the assistance with ADLs and IADLs provided by services and by carers. Consistent with the existing literature, it suggests that people living in the community rarely receive assistance from services at an intensity similar to that provided in long-term care settings, and that the majority of their help is provided by carers. It also shows that some carers continued to be involved in direct assistance, even though the person for whom they cared had been admitted into long-term care.

Just over half the sample were reported to be continent. A third were reported to be incontinent of urine. In the first NISW study, incontinence was associated with admission to residential care (Levin et al, 1989). We found that, although proportionally more people in long-term care were doubly incontinent, it was not statistically significant. It may be that better continence management and the wider availability of continence aids has made it easier to maintain in the community people with dementia who are incontinent.

We also considered the impact of behavioural changes. Along with hallucinations, delusions and depressive features, they are generally considered to form part of the non-cognitive features, or neuropsychiatric symptoms, of dementia (Allen and Burns, 1995). They have been defined as including aggression, activity disturbances (such as excessive walking), eating behaviour (such as decreased or increased food intake), disturbances of diurnal rhythm (such as sleep disturbance), sexual behaviour (such as disinhibition in public) and other miscellaneous disturbances (Hope and Patel, 1993).

While behavioural changes are not experienced by everyone with dementia, they are particularly problematic in that they can cause significant distress both to the sufferers themselves and to their carers. They are often one of the main reasons for a person being admitted into long-term care (Burns, 1996).

The 'gold standard' for measuring the type and frequency of behavioural change is observation (Hope and Patel, 1993). However, this approach is not always feasible and there are a number of questionnaires designed to be completed by carers and staff which include items designed to measure the nature and extent of behavioural problems in dementia (Greene et al, 1982; Nolan and Grant,

1992). We asked carers and proxy informants a series of questions about the older person's behaviour and positive personality traits (Levin et al, 1989). (The full list is recorded in Appendix 3.)

Almost all the older people in the sample were reported to have at least one positive trait and one trying behaviour. Out of a maximum possible score of 8, study participants scored a mean of 5 positive traits (SD 2); out of a maximum of 9 trying behaviours, the mean score was 4 (SD 2). The mean rank of positive personality trait and trying behaviour scores did not differ significantly between men and women, nor did the severity of their dementia as measured by the OBS.

Contrary to our initial expectations, the mean rank of trying behaviours and positive personality traits did not differ significantly between people living in residential or nursing homes, hospital or in the community at Time One. It is possible that these results are an artefact of sample selection. Within the nursing homes and hospital wards in the SSD, there would have been people with very severe behavioural problems who were not referred to the SSD during the period over which we collected referrals. Nevertheless, the absence of any difference between the people in long-term care and those living in the community does contrast with the other measures we used to compare participants across settings, where we found strong associations between severity of dementia, depression and functional disability and living in long-term care.

Table 7.3 shows that the mean rank of reported positive traits was lowest for people with co-resident carers and the mean rank of trying behaviours was highest, although the latter was not significant at the 5% level.

We cannot discount the possibility of over- or under-reporting between different types of informant. In order to consider the influence of informant type and sampling source, we compared participants' trying behaviours and positive traits scores with those obtained in the respite care study. This was a study of 287 people with dementia who had current co-resident carers. The sample had been recruited mainly from specialist secondary healthcare sources (Levin et al, 1994). The observed distributions of trying behaviour scores did not

Table 7.3: Reported trying behaviours and positive traits by informant

Type of informant	Mean rank of trying behaviours	Mean rank of positive traits	Valid n
Co-resident carer	80.80	48.46	27
Non-resident carer	68.54	65.18	40
Former carer	58.95	71.34	32
Proxy	57.39	76.48	32
Significance (n)	χ^2=7.2; 3 df; p=0.06	χ^2=9.0; 3 df; p=0.03	(131)

differ between the two data sets (K-S Z=0.70; p=0.7), but there was a significant difference between the distribution of the positive trait scores (K-S Z=-1.40; p=0.03). Participants in this study were rated more positively than those in the respite care study. However, when proxy informants were excluded from the analysis, the distribution of the reported positive scores did not appear to differ between the two sets of carers (K-S Z =0.4298; p= 0.99).

The difference between co-resident carers and other informants raises two possibilities. The first is that co-resident carers may have more opportunities to observe the behaviour of the person with dementia. The second is that extended contact may have negative consequences for the way in which the personality traits of the cared for person are perceived. It is interesting that former carers, who had less contact with the older person and were giving less assistance with ADLs and IADLs than current carers, produced similar scores to those reported by proxies.

Other data also suggested that there were associations between the two scores and the amount of caring tasks that were undertaken. In terms of those who were currently caring, there was a positive correlation between trying behaviours and the number of ADLs with they were giving assistance (Spearman's ρ=0.4; p=0.000) and with GHQ score (0.26; p=0.02) There were negative correlations between positive traits and assistance with ADLs (Spearman's ρ=-0.33, p=0.003) and GHQ (Spearman's ρ=-0.29; p=0.008). It is possible that giving more direct physical care presents greater opportunities for disagreements between carer and older person.

The mean rank of positive traits was higher for people whose carers reported feeling close to them (U=291.0; p=0.0001), but the mean rank of trying behaviours did not differ significantly between the carers who felt close to the person for whom they cared and those who did not.

Non-resident carers did report problems with night disturbance, for instance if the older person telephoned thinking that it was daytime. Unsurprisingly, however, this was more of an issue for co-resident carers. Co-resident carers reported that their sleep had been interrupted for an average of 14 nights in the previous month, compared with once for non-resident carers (F=34.0; p=0.00). Older people cared for by proxy informants, who were almost always paid staff in residential or nursing homes, were generally reported to sleep well.

Former co-resident and current co-resident carers were much more likely to report that they had been hit by the older person since the onset of the symptoms associated with dementia than were former and current non resident carers (χ^2=11.1; 1 df; p=0.0008). Just three proxy informants said that they had been hit by the older person.

Eighty per cent of current co-resident carers reported that they sometimes or often lost their temper with the person for whom they cared, compared with half the non-resident carers and less than a fifth of the former carers (χ^2=11.1; 1 df; p=0.004). Similarly, six of the eight carers who admitted that they had shaken or smacked the older person were current co-resident carers.

In summary, it was co-resident carers in the sample who appeared to experience the greatest impact from the problems associated with behavioural change. In particular, they were the group who reported most problems with night disturbance and aggression.

Comparisons between long-term care settings

Chapter 8 suggests that the rates of placement in nursing care were lower than the national average. The numbers of people living in nursing and residential homes at Time One was too small to permit statistical analyses comparing the two subgroups, but the proportion of people with severe dementia and depression was similar in both settings. On the basis of the carers' and proxy informants' answers, we did not find any differences between residential and nursing home residents in terms of whether they had a coexisting health problem such as diabetes or arthritis. However, residents in nursing care at Time One were more likely to have died by Time Two. It may be that these findings reflect the increasingly blurred distinction between residential and nursing homes that is reported by private and voluntary sector home owners (Royal Commission on Long Term Care, 1999). Some proxy informants suggested that people had been assessed as needing residential care rather than nursing care for cost reasons. One proxy informant working in a dual registration home exclaimed:

"It's care on the cheap!"

Of the people admitted into long-term care over the course of the study, we found only eight for whom the NHS was reported to be making a contribution to the costs of their care. Three of these had died by Time Two and none lived in the metropolitan borough. The longstanding variation in the types of long-term provision, which means that people with similar needs living in different parts of the country can receive different forms of care, is one of the factors contributing to the sense of unfairness about current long-term care funding arrangements. The development of a long-term care charter is part of the Fair Access to Care initiative outlined in *Modernising social services*

(Secretary of State for Health, 1998).

Survival analyses examining entry into long-term care

In this chapter so far, comparisons between people remaining at home and people entering long-term care have been made using Time One data. As we have explained, although the proportion of people living at home declined over the course of the study, almost a third of the original 141 participants were still at home by Time Two. One of the ways of handling censored data, that is, cases for which the event under investigation has not yet occurred (in this case, entry to long-term care), is to use survival analyses.

Survival analyses were conducted on data on service receipt, the SSD in which the person lived, access to a carer and severity of cognitive impairment at assessment. In this context, scores on the NISW Noticeable Problems (Levin et al, 1989) were used in preference to those on the OBS from the BAS (Macdonald et al, 1982) because they had been obtained nearer to the assessment. Long-term care was defined as a move to residential, nursing or long-term hospital care with no planned or provisional date of discharge. The analysis excluded nine people already living in long-term care at the time of referral but included 19 people living at home when they were referred who died during the study period. Of these, four people admitted to hospital for medical reasons a few days before death and one person who died during respite care were treated as having remained in the community. The others, who had spent at least six weeks away from their home address prior to death (mean number of days 307, SD 215), were treated as having entered long-term care. This approach is consistent with that adopted by Hope and colleagues (1998).

Severity of cognitive impairment

The main predictor of entry into long-term care was severity of cognitive impairment. This is shown in Figure 7.1, which plots the Kaplan–Meier survival estimates for people whose scores on the NISW Noticeable Problems showed they had mild, moderate or severe cognitive impairment. The survival plot shows three lines, each starting at the value of '1' on the vertical axis, representing 100% of the people living in the community or in hospital at the time of their referral. Each line represents a score on the NISW Noticeable Problems. The bottom line shows scores of 5 and 6 which indicate severe cognitive impairment. The middle line represents people with moderate cognitive impairment (scores of 3-4), while the top line indicates mild cognitive impairment (scores of 1-2).

The figure shows how, as time passed, the proportion living in the community diminished as more and more of the older people entered long-term care. Those whose scores on the NISW Noticeable Problems suggested that they had severe cognitive impairment entered long-term care more rapidly (estimated mean time seven months) than those with moderate and mild cognitive impairment (estimated mean time 13 and 16 months respectively).

The analyses showed that the assumption of proportional hazards was true. In other words, entry rates to long-term care were proportional

over time among participants at different stages of cognitive impairment. Despite the varying rates of entry into long-term care among the moderately cognitively impaired group, shown by the way that the curve zigzags between the severe and mild curves, it does not cross either line. Log Rank, Breslow and Tarone–Ware tests all show that the survival curve for severe cognitive impairment was significantly steeper than the curves for moderate ($p \leq 0.04$) and mild cognitive impairment ($p \leq 0.0003$) but the tests did not show a difference between the moderate and mild cognitive impairment curves ($p \geq 0.29$).

Impact of having a carer

People whose scores on the NISW Noticeable Problems suggested that they had mild or moderate cognitive impairment were about half as likely to have entered long-term care if they had a spouse or a daughter carer in comparison with those cared for by 'others' (that is, all those carers who were not the spouse or daughter of the person for whom they cared) or those without a carer.

Figure 7.1: Proportion of older people living at home between referral to SSD and Time Two by severity of cognitive impairment at assessment

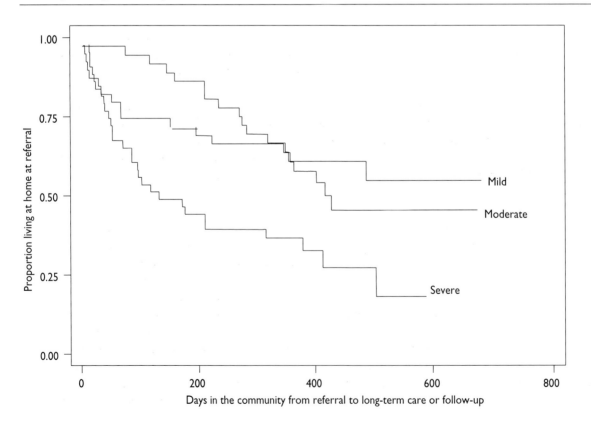

Table 7.4: Cox regression survival analysis: percentage of study participants entering long-term care

	% entering long-term care	Adjusted odds ratio	95% CL	*p*	*n*
Home care					
Yes	47	1			59
No	67	2.48	1.43 to 4.31	0.001	61
Day care					
Yes	33	1			52
No	76	5.96	2.79 to 12.7	0.000	68
Short stay					
Yes	48	1			25
No	60	0.57	0.25 to 1.31	0.19	95
Study area					
Metropolitan	68	1			53
London	69	0.86	0.44 to 1.67	0.66	26
County	37	0.63	0.33 to 1.23	0.18	41
Spouse or daughter care					
Yes	43	1			58
No	71	3.36	0.9 to 12.3	0.07	62
Access to any carer					
No	87	1			23
Yes	47	0.41	0.14 to 1.23	0.11	97

Interaction terms*	Cognitive impairment						
	Mild	Mod	Sev				
Spouse or daughter	16	38	67	3.28	1.64 to 6.55	0.001	58
Other carer	37	50	63	1.71	0.98 to 2.97	0.059	39
No carer	62	75	100	1.36	0.79 to 2.32	0.265	23
All (*n*)	(58)						120

*The nested hierarchical model tests for interaction effects (that is, whether severity of cognitive impairment has a differential impact upon the three types of care arrangement). The interaction terms are as follows:

(Spouse or daughter carer) x (cognitive impairment) = 0 for those without a spouse or daughter carer. For those with a spouse or daughter carer, scores vary in accordance with the severity of cognitive impairment (0: mild, 1: moderate, 2: severe). (Other carer) x (cognitive impairment) = 0 for those with spouse or daughter carer or no carer. For those with other carers, 0-2 as above. (No carer) x (cognitive impairment) = 0 for those with any carer. For those without a carer, 0-2 as above.

The increased probability of mildly and moderate cognitively impaired people with spouse and daughter carers remaining at home is confirmed by the results from a Cox regression survival analysis which are presented in Table 7.4. The analysis adjusts the odds of entering long-term care to take into account the services received and area differences while testing for a differential impact of severity of cognitive impairment on access to a spouse or daughter carer, having another carer, and not having a carer.

Using the adjusted odds from the survival analysis presented in Table 7.4, the estimated probability of entering long-term care at Time Two for people with a spouse or daughter carer increased from 16% of those who were mildly cognitively impaired to 38% of those with moderate cognitive impairment and to 67% of those with severe cognitive impairment. At the same time, it shows that the increased probability of people with spouse or daughter carers remaining at home did not hold good for people with severe cognitive impairment.

Impact of the receipt of community services

Table 7.4 also shows that 47% of home care users were in long-term care at follow-up, compared with 67% of non users. In so far as day care was concerned, 33% of users had entered long-term care at follow-up compared with 76% of non-attenders. The use of short-stay care did not increase the likelihood of admission into long-term care. This is consistent with results from the respite care study, in which this variable was excluded from the final model of factors significantly predicting entry into long-term care (Levin et al, 1994). Although a smaller proportion of people in the county council went into long-term care, it would appear that this was a function of the higher proportion of people with spouse or daughter carers and day care attenders in the county than in the other SSDs, and was not an area difference.

Although the analyses were able to control for differences in the levels of provision of home care and day care within the study areas and the severity of the participants' cognitive impairment, some potentially confounding factors remain. These centre on whether the apparent effects of a service might actually be explained by other differences between those who received it and those who did not (for instance, a co-existing physical illness).

Funding for long-term care

The proportion of people entering long-term care over the course of the study highlighted the importance of how their care was to be funded. Dissatisfaction with funding arrangements for long-term care was an issue raised by spontaneously by many carers, and we have reported their comments in more detail elsewhere (Moriarty and Webb, 1998).

At Time One, around a third of the people in residential and nursing care were entirely self-funding. This proportion is similar to that found overall among people living in long-term care. Of the 482,250 people living in long-term care, some 320,000 are publicly financed (Royal Commission on Long Term Care, 1999, p 9).

We had originally wondered whether self-funding people would have fewer needs than those who were funded by the SSD. In the event, self-funding and SSD-funded participants did not appear to differ. The explanation probably lies in the fact that they had all been *assessed* as meeting the SSD's criteria for entry to long-term care.

Although the variation in the period for which people require long-term care is well known, it has been suggested that most SSDs do not know how long older people stay in residential or nursing homes or for how long they receive domiciliary services. This makes it difficult for them to estimate spending and service needs for the future (SSI, 1999).

Nearly all self-funding residents used the sale of housing assets to fund their care (Moriarty and Webb, 1998) and so they required SSD funding for a period until their property was sold. By Time Two, seven people had spent down their capital to below the £10,000 limit operating at the time. Among the survivors, the number of people fully funding their own care was 13. The increase in the number of people living in long-term care at Time Two meant that the proportion of fully or partially local authority funded residents in long-term care had risen to 87%.

Six of the study participants had 'preserved rights' to DSS support because they had entered long-term care before April 1993. By Time Two, over 80% (*n*=29) of the 35 people in residential care at Time One were still there; one person had been transferred to nursing care and five people had died. Of the 14 people living in nursing homes, six had died by Time Two and the remainder were still living there. This lends support to the suggestion that SSDs appear to be gradually accruing responsibilities for funding increasing proportions of people in residential and nursing care (Edwards and Kenny, 1997). This, in turn, will affect the sums that are available to support 'new' clients.

Views of people with dementia about long-term care

If the likelihood is high that people with dementia will move into long-term care, then we need to consider how this fits in with their own preferences. It has been suggested that, within society as a whole, the idea of living in a residential or nursing home has become more acceptable. Many people may prefer to live in some form of long-term care than be looked after by their family (PPP Lifetime Care, 1996).

This study suggested that people with dementia held differing views about the prospect of moving to a residential or nursing home. In Chapter 3, we reported that some people with dementia associated their depression with entry into long-term care. Mrs Guy was one of these:

"You're asking me at a bad time. Why am I sent here? I'm not ill. I'm used to being by myself. I feel as though I'm being expelled. My son said I was here because I'm not very well but I'm not ill. I feel as though I've done something wrong. Why am I here?"

Case example

Mrs Patrick lived alone at Time One. She had no immediate family but was visited by a home care worker, "a nice young woman, always sees that I'm fed. She'll make me my dinner and leaves me my tea." On being asked her hopes for the future in the BAS interview, she replied: "To stay here and die in my own home." This was not a prospect that made her sad: "I'm always happy. I'm lonely but I'm not because I've got my home." By Time Two, home care had increased to three times a day, including help from an agency at the weekend. When asked the same questions, her replies were strikingly consistent with those she had given at Time One: "I am stopping here in my own little home. I love my home!"

In contrast, others who had made the transition were pleased. Mr Samuel lived in a residential home. As a former chef, he was delighted to be able to help at meal times:

"I like it here. I feel safe."

There were also some examples of good practice where people living in long-term care had opportunities to maintain the life-style they had led when living at home.

Case example

At Time One, Mrs Wilfred lived on her own during the week but stayed with her daughter and son-in-law at the weekend. By the Time Two interviews she had moved into a residential home. By a happy coincidence, she was able to re-establish contact with some former work colleagues also living in the home. On the day she was interviewed, she was wearing a bright pink jumper. When asked how she was feeling, she joked, "I'm in the pink!" She still continued to spend her weekends with her daughter and son-in-law.

Carers' attitudes towards long-term care

It has been suggested that the emphasis on community care has led to residential or nursing care being perceived as second best when, in fact, carers may believe it is the right setting (MacDonald et al, 1996). Few studies have interviewed those who have ceased to care at more than one point in time. Pushkar Gold and colleagues (1995) found that, by the time former carers were interviewed for a second time, they generally felt satisfied with their decision and were pleased with the home that had been selected. We also found that many carers had gradually adjusted to ceasing to care and had come to terms with what had happened. Consistent with the findings of Simpson and colleagues (1995), there was also evidence that many carers continued to be involved in decision making. For instance, many had made arrangements to attend review meetings, although the person for whom they cared was living in a residential or nursing home.

Case example

Mr Jacobs, an only son, used to visit his mother daily. His mother was admitted to a residential home because her mobility had become so restricted after a fall. At Time One, he felt guilty that he had not encouraged his mother to accept help from the SSD sooner: "I wish I had done something sooner [about contacting services]. If I had, maybe she wouldn't have fallen and had to go into a home." In the interval between Times One and Two his partner developed a terminal illness and died. He described his relief at knowing that his mother was safe during his partner's terminal illness. His advice to others in his position was: "Don't fight it! Let your relative go into a home!"

Assessment and care management

Care management in the UK has mainly developed since the final implementation of the 1990 NHS and Community Care Act (Challis et al, 1998). While Challis and colleagues (1997) reported positive outcomes for people with dementia in Lewisham where an experimental intensive care management was in operation, they suggested that it was unlikely that all people with dementia would be able to receive this sort of service. It has been suggested that three main types of care management seem to be in operation across SSDs (Edwards, 1996, p 122):

- *administrative:* supplying information and advice;
- *coordinating:* arranging a single service or range of straightforward services, continuing support not required;
- *intensive:* combining the planning and coordination of services with a therapeutic, supportive role.

Our study was not designed to give a detailed examination of the types of care management that were in operation in the study SSDs. However, comments from the carers and data on service utilisation patterns suggested that most participants received the second type of care management.

Once started, the use of services rarely ceased; rather, services were used incrementally, either because their intensity was increased or because they were supplemented by more intensive forms of care. About two thirds of participants appeared to have had their care reviewed between Times One and Two, but some carers remained unclear as to who was undertaking the planning and coordination of services. When asked about which professionals she had seen since the first interview, one carer replied wearily:

"[I've] seen so many people last year. So many people ring me up [that] it is difficult to know which is which!"

It is a comment that was to be echoed by many carers, both current and former. Mrs Howard, who cared for her father, wanted better communication between care managers, families and providers:

"It takes you a while to pick up their jargon. [Father] went into The Oaks [for a short stay] without having an assessment although we and [social worker] had told them he had senile dementia. They hadn't got a clue. They were absolutely useless!"

Discussion

Data showing the different care paths taken by study participants have important implications for improving assessment and care management practices and the commissioning of social care services for people with dementia.

Almost all the participants had been assessed by a qualified social worker. Just over a quarter of study participants were offered long-term care as a result of the assessment. Of the remainder, very few people entered long-term care in the five or six month interval between being assessed and Time One. This suggested that assessors were arranging durable and sustainable care packages which rarely broke down.

Much of the published work on services since the implementation of the community care changes has looked at management processes and strategic change. There has been less on the skills required by practitioners. These results suggest that future research could examine the relationship between assessors' professional backgrounds, their levels of experience and the degree to which these are reflected in the outcomes of their assessments and the sustainability of the care packages they arrange.

All in all, there is evidence that the community care changes have led to a reduction in the numbers of people in long-term care (Royal Commission on Long Term Care, 1999). Within the study SSDs, it appeared that long-term care was targeted on people with more severe dementia and with higher levels of functional disability, as measured by the assistance they received with ADLs.

While the increased risk of entry to long-term care among people with dementia is well known, the study offers new evidence suggesting that, within this group, rates of entry do differ. Over an 18-month period between referral and Time Two, they were quickest among people with severe cognitive impairment. The mean interval between referral and entry to long-term care among study participants with severe cognitive impairment was almost a year less than that for people with mild cognitive impairment.

It is becoming increasingly clear that there is considerable variation in the lengths of time for which people use community and long-term care services. The design of the study has enabled us to contribute to this debate. The number of people in long-term care at Time One who were still there at Time Two adds to the growing body of evidence that SSDs appear to be gradually accruing responsibilities for funding increasing proportions of people in residential and nursing care.

The evidence on the contribution made by carers in delaying entry to long-term care was consistent with the existing literature that the support offered by spouses and daughters is greater than that afforded by other types of carer, or where there is no carer. However, the study adds to our understanding by demonstrating how the impact of severe dementia is such that even the most committed of carers may reach a point at which they feel unable to carry on caring. Former carers and staff working in long-term care settings can testify to the intense feelings of distress and guilt experienced by many carers when the person for whom they care is admitted to long-term care. In the process of arranging admissions to long-term care, carers need two types of support. First, they need the affirmation that the event does not invalidate the contribution they have made in the past. Second, they need to feel confident they will be allowed to continue to play a role in future care, if this is in accordance with their wishes and those of the person with dementia.

In terms of the people with dementia, the study adds to the existing and worrying evidence that depression is under-recognised in social care settings (Banerjee and Macdonald, 1996; Banerjee et al, 1996; Schneider et al, 1997b). Their comments showed that the concept of 'home' was important to them and that many felt a sense of loss as a result of moving into long-term care. Although very few people with dementia knew where they were in terms of the location or the address, they were aware that they were not at home. Here, it may be helpful to view disorientation as a continuum. It is also important to find ways of making the process of adjustment to long-term care easier. There were examples of study participants who had made a successful transition. Future work could examine the ways in which staff practices and the culture in long-term care settings could contribute to this process.

The last two chapters have described the community and long-term care services received by participants. The next chapter examines the costs of the care that they received.

8

Costs of packages of care for older people with dementia

Ann Netten, Angela Hallam and Jane Knight

Key points

- This chapter explains what was involved in calculating the costs of care packages.

- Location was a key influence on costs.

- When accommodation costs and living expenses are included, the mean weekly cost of community services was similar to that of residential care.

- Local authority purchased care dominated in all three areas.

- 'Lifetime use' of short-term breaks and the high contribution to package costs of short-term breaks in hospital are discussed.

Introduction

The level and types of care package being received by older people with dementia and their carers have been described in the two previous chapters. This chapter examines the implications of these service packages for the costs of care. The chapter starts by describing the underlying principles of costing and the estimation process, before outlining the results in terms of costs of services and packages received. For the purposes here, the focus is on the initial package that was put into place immediately after the case was assessed.

Principles

The theoretical and pragmatic basis for estimating the opportunity costs of care packages has been described in detail elsewhere (Netten and Beecham, 1993). The process of estimation depends on, and has implications for, the way in which cost information can and should be used. Integrating these issues, Knapp (1993) has identified the basic principles of applied costs research and has summarised them in four 'rules':

- comprehensiveness;
- ensuring that like is compared with like;
- identifying and exploring cost variations;
- integrating costs with information on outcomes.

The first rule, that costs should be measured comprehensively, is particularly pertinent when identifying the costs of packages that in some cases include residential care. In order to ensure that the second rule is adhered to (that like is compared with like), it is important that the costs of community-based packages include accommodation and living expenses which are automatically included in the costs of residential based care. With respect to the third rule (that variations in costs are identified and explored), local costs need to be used, as local decision making will be affected by local circumstances reflected in the relative costs of different services. Variation in the cost of care packages would also be expected to reflect the relative needs of older people and their carers. Here we are simply describing the cost implications of the care packages put into place, so outcomes and costs are not related to an individual.

Methodology

The data on service receipt at Time One were collected primarily during the financial year 1995/96 so the unit costs were estimated for or adjusted to reflect 1995/96 costs. The comprehensive costs of caring for older people include the cost of local authority provision, the cost of independently provided services, the cost of health services and the cost of accommodation and living expenses. Different approaches were required for each of these.

Local authority provision

Each of the SSDs had estimates of the unit costs of many in-house services. Methods of calculation differ, however, and accounts information may conceal costs to other agencies (Allen and Beecham, 1993). In order to measure costs consistently and comprehensively across the three local authorities taking part in the study, it was important to understand how unit costs had been calculated, and to supplement elements where necessary.

In the case of home care services, the basis of unit cost information supplied was checked to ensure that all the essential elements had been included and that allowance had been made for time spent travelling and so on. In one authority adjustments were made to unit costs used as guides within the SSD to allow for time spent on supporting activities rather than directly with clients. In each authority differential rates were applied reflecting the time that the service was delivered (weekdays daytime, evenings, weekends and so on). The authority rates reflected expected regional variation, with the metropolitan borough costing £6.98 per hour, the county £8.40 per hour and the London borough £11.50 per hour in daytime hours on weekdays.

One local authority provided considerable detail on the costs of home care including the proportion of contact to non-contact hours. Seventy-seven per cent of home care workers' time was spent in direct contact. This was slightly lower than found in previous work reported in Netten and Dennett (1996) and converts to a ratio of 1:0.295 compared with 1:0.22 currently used to estimate national costs. This direction of difference would be expected, given the characteristics of the authority. Direct

overheads, excluding travel but including management, supplies and services, added 20% to wage costs, and indirect overheads reflecting support service and capital added a further 20%. Although overheads would be expected to be somewhat higher than nationally, these are considerably higher than estimates currently used (16% for all overheads).

The only other in-house services provided were day and residential care. The authorities supplied running costs for each of the local authority residential homes and day centres which had been used by study clients. The information was broken down into different categories so that it was clear which elements had been included. Capital and equipment values were taken from Netten and Dennett (1996). Although these figures relate to new-build information, and therefore reflect a situation not entirely appropriate for the residential and day units used in the study, such details ensured that capital was not underestimated, and that the estimates were comparable across the three local authorities. Regional adjustments were made using the Building Cost Information Service Index. When annuitising the value of capital, HM Treasury recommends that, when publicly provided capital is for a service that is traded on the open market, 8% should be used. As most residential care is now provided by the independent sector, this was taken as the most appropriate rate. (If capital is discounted at 6%, the costs of local authority residential care would be 5% lower than presented here, that is, between £13 and £15 per week less.) Day care capital costs were also discounted at 8%. Managing agency overheads were assumed to be 5% of the total cost of both residential (Audit Commission, 1993) and day care.

Where a residential home provides services to non-residents, these elements need to be teased out from other running expenses and costed independently. Day care, for example, is often provided within a residential unit, and it is important to identify the resources associated with this service because the costs of day care are likely to form a substantial contribution to total service package costs. Residential units that provided day care were identified and normally found to have separate accounts for residential provision and day care. Not all running costs were apportioned, but it was possible to make estimates, based on the advice of contacts (finance or service managers) at the participating local authorities.

For the most part, short-term breaks were costed on the basis of the average daily cost of the home in which the older person stayed. In one home it was possible to identify the additional costs of providing short-term breaks as the staffing was separately identified. In this case, short-term breaks were 10% more costly per week than long-term care.

Meals-on-wheels costs were based on locally provided estimates with additions made for overhead costs where appropriate.

The information about social work input or other professional input during the assessment process was too insufficient for it to be included in the cost of assessment in the cost of the package. The focus of the study was on the experiences of users and carers. As was explained in Chapter 4, the carers and proxy informants did not necessarily know the full extent of other professional contacts at assessment, and collecting this information would have required considerable tracking of service contacts via client records which was never part of the study's remit.

Independently provided services

The costs of independently provided services to the local authority are the prices charged. Price information was collected for home care, sitting agencies and day care. For the present purposes, it was assumed that contract prices covered costs and that there was no subsidy for voluntary provision. Where block contracts were in operation, advice was taken from the local authority in converting this to an estimated cost per case. In cases where the information was not available, the price of the nearest equivalent service in that authority was used.

The agreed price of placement in independent residential and nursing homes was used with top-up payments included where applicable. In two of the authorities, the price excluding top-up was the same for all residential and for all nursing homes. In the London authority, individual prices were contracted with homes.

Health service provision

The majority of service provision identified was social care, which is the main focus of interest here. Ideally, we would include comprehensive health service inputs, reflecting local cost variations. In practice, limited information was available about service receipt or local prices, so unit costs from Netten and Dennett (1996) were used for district nurse and CPN visits, GP contacts, day hospital services and inpatient stays (including both short-term and admissions for treatment). For the most part, national average figures were used for all health services, so variations in health service costs reflect variation in service receipt. The effect of allowing for the higher costs associated with London on inpatient care (for both short-term and medical care) and on day care costs are also reported. An inflator of 1.22 was used to reflect the higher costs of providing these services in London (Akehurst et al, 1991).

Where possible, information about hospital costs distinguished whether the older person was admitted to a psychiatric hospital rather than for emergency or planned medical treatment. It was not possible, however, to distinguish between the costs of short-term breaks and admissions for planned operations, as information on hospital expenditure does not distinguish between the types of care provided. Necessarily, therefore, short-term breaks costs are likely to be overestimates and planned operations underestimates of actual service costs.

It was not felt appropriate to ask for detailed information about service receipt for chiropody, occupational therapy, physiotherapy, health visitor, optician, dentist, psychologist, geriatrician and old age psychiatrists. Information was collected, however, about whether people received the service. The most frequently received services of this uncosted element of the package were those of a chiropodist and optician. For those for whom information was known, 61% of older people receiving community-based packages were seeing a chiropodist and 48% an optician. The cost of these services would not have added substantially to the package costs as it is rare for people to visit a chiropodist more than once every six weeks, or opticians more than annually. A six-weekly visit from the chiropodist would increase the average weekly cost by less than £4.

Estimation of costs of short-term breaks

Short-term breaks were provided in local authority and independent homes, in hospital and, in one case, in the older person's home. At Time One, carers or proxies were asked when the older person first used short-term breaks, how many sessions had been received since they first started and, for up to three specified venues, the number of stays and average length of stay. In order to estimate weekly package costs of short-term breaks, it was necessary to draw on Time Two interviews which identified the number and length of stays during the study period. Package costs were estimated as the total cost of stays divided by the number of weeks in the study period (from Time One until admission to long-term care, death or Time Two interview). Admission to long-term care was taken as the date of admission to a home or hospital after which the person died or did not return home, whether or not the original intention had been that this should be a long-term placement.

There is a lack of information in the literature about the regularity and cost of long-term packages of care. Two issues are of interest: first, how much do short-term breaks contribute to package costs, both for those who receive it and more generally for people with dementia receiving community-based care? Second, for those who have used short-term breaks, what are the lifetime costs of receiving the service? As data were collected about the receipt of short-term breaks both before and during the study period, it was possible to address both these issues.

Additional services received in residential care

No information was collected about other services received while in residential care at Time One. Previous research (Knapp et al, 1989; Netten and Topan, 1996) indicates that 5% can be added to the costs of care to allow for all other services (including local authority day care and community health services). This has been used as a proxy for additional service consumption for those in residential and nursing home care. It is possible that

in this context this is an overestimate: not all potential additional services are being costed in community-based service packages in this study, and results at Time Two suggested that individuals in this study were receiving few additional services.

Domestic accommodation

For clients living in owner-occupied households, a capital valuation of the property was estimated for the first quarter of 1996 (Halifax Building Society, 1996). It was possible to use region-specific average market figures, and to distinguish between houses and flats/maisonettes. Figures were annuitised at 8% over the average 60-year life expectancy of a property.

Valuations of local authority property were taken from government-produced statistics (DoE, 1994, Table 10.19). These were based on mortgages to first-time purchasers who were local authority sitting tenants in 1993, and the prices were uprated to 1995-96 price levels using the Department of the Environment Public Building Work Output Price Index. The percentage discount on sales was 50% in both 1993-94 and 1994-95 (Housing Data and Statistics Division, DoE, personal communication), so average prices were doubled to arrive at the appropriate market valuation. A subsidy element per dwelling, including supervision and management and repairs and maintenance, was calculated using *CIPFA Housing Revenue Account Statistics 1992-93* (CIPFA, 1992) inflated to 1995-96 price levels.

Sheltered housing costs were based on estimates by Netten and Dennett (1996) derived from a survey of sheltered accommodation (McCafferty, 1994). These costs covered the capital costs, maintenance costs, management support and warden services. The London borough was assumed to be 15% more costly.

Living expenses

The Family Expenditure Survey (FES), published by the Central Statistical Office, provides information on average amounts spent on essential items (such as housing, basic provisions, household bills and travel) by various sizes and compositions of household, and at different income levels. Client and carer household income details collected at interview were compared with FES data for the relevant status and composition of the household (including age), and a weekly expenditure figure was calculated. When the older person was living in owner-occupied accommodation, expenditure was taken to include housing expenses; for older people who do not have mortgage commitments, these expenses consist of repairs and maintenance. For all other groups, expenditure excluding housing expenses was used to estimate living expenses.

People who are resident in residential or nursing homes also incur some personal expenses (such as clothes and toiletries) which are not covered by the home's fees or expenditure. The DSS personal allowance (£13 per week) provided for publicly funded residents was used as a proxy for this expenditure.

Results

Costs of services

Table 8.1 shows the level of service receipt, the average and the median cost for those in receipt of any services and for whom there was sufficient information to estimate costs (120). Local authority purchased or provided services are distinguished from health service receipt.

A high proportion of people were admitted to residential or nursing home care as a result of their assessment. The range of costs of this option depended on whether people had been admitted to residential or nursing home care. The weekly costs reported in Table 8.1 reflect the proportions of people admitted to local authority homes (18%), independent residential homes (53%) and nursing homes (29%). Compared with the national picture

Table 8.1: Level of service receipt and cost for those receiving services at Time One

	Number of people receiving services	Mean weekly cost per person (£)	Median weekly cost per person (£)
Local authority provided and purchased services			
Residential or nursing home care	48	286.09	298.55
Home care	48	41.88	39.00
Day care	33	78.66	53.60
Short-term care	12	37.26	28.93
Meals-on-wheels	13	8.09	5.66
Home-based carer support	7	58.65	25.20
Community services total	69	80.71	59.34
NHS provision			
Day hospital	13	205.25	174.00
Inpatient care*	8	61.15	17.54
Short-term care	9	146.68	129.31
GP consultations	44	5.05	3.62
District nurse	10	27.35	25.96
Community psychiatric nurse	8	10.06	3.83
Health services total	57	86.56	24.60
All services total	**120**	**200.31**	**226.98**

*Temporary stays only. Excludes one person who was in hospital before assessment with no planned date of discharge at a weekly cost of £798.00. Including an allowance for higher costs in London, mean weekly costs of day hospital would be £219.15; short-term care £158.57; all services £202.71. The median costs of day hospital, short-term care and all services would be unchanged.

of admissions of all publicly funded older people, a lower proportion was admitted to nursing homes (42% nationally), and a higher proportion to local authority homes (9% nationally) (Bebbington et al, 1996).

Home care was the most frequently received service for those receiving a community-based package. The cost of home care depended on the time of day it was received, the level of service receipt and the local authority level of unit costs. The skewed distribution indicated by the difference between the median and the mean reflect variation between the authorities. Within each authority, the mean and the median values were within £10 of each other. As would be expected, home care costs in the London borough were higher (on average £69 per week). The average weekly cost was £40 in the county and £30 in the metropolitan borough.

The few cases that received sitting services for the most part received relatively few hours. The high average cost of this service reflected one very costly case where a sleeping-in service was being provided five nights per week in the metropolitan borough at a weekly cost of £200. The median cost is a better guide to the costs of sitting service receipt.

The costs of day care services were similarly affected by location. Most people who attended day care visited homes for older people or day centres. The median weekly cost of those attending day care was £54 per week. One person attended day care seven days per week in a very costly local authority home with estimated costs close to £300 per week. Nearly a third of those using day care services attended day hospital, reflecting the characteristics of this client group. (Only one person was attending both day care and day hospital.) The unit cost is much higher for day hospitals, and this is reflected in the median cost of £174 per week for those attending day hospital.

For both short-term breaks and day care, it is important to bear in mind that an accurate and area-specific cost of health service provision has not been possible. We can be reasonably confident from previous work, however, that hospital costs do exceed the costs of local authority purchased and provided provision.

As would be expected, the healthcare service received by most people is the GP. In the three months prior to the interview at Time One, over half of those receiving community services had seen their GP at an average weekly cost of £5. Community nurses, in contrast, were rarely seen regularly by this group. Inpatient care costs reflect the weekly average of costs of stays over the preceding three months.

Table 8.1 summarises (for those people for whom all service costs are known) the costs of services for those receiving community-based local authority purchased and provided services and for those receiving health services. These are clearly lower than the costs of residential based care but, as has been advised above, it is important to compare like with like. In order to do this, it is important to include the costs of accommodation and living expenses in the costs of community-based packages.

Costs of short-term breaks costs

The lack of information about the use and costs of short-term breaks was identified above. Although relatively few people were receiving the service, the data allow us to explore some aspects of patterns of service receipt and associated costs. Three perspectives are explored: the level of receipt and costs for those who received the service during the study period; the impact of the service on package costs; and the lifetime costs of short-term breaks receipt.

Although 27 people were reported as receiving short-term breaks at Time One, just 20 people received short-term breaks during the study period (between the first and second interviews or death). There was considerable variation in the costs of short-term care, reflecting the length of each stay, the frequency of stays and the characteristics of the venue. Short-term breaks that took place in hospital are listed separately in Table 8.1 to reflect the most important source of variation: the location. (One person appears in both sections as she received short-term breaks both in hospital and in residential care.)

During the study period, people stayed on average 11 days per stay (median 14 days) in hospital and 10 days per stay in residential or nursing homes (median seven days). They stayed on average twice in residential or nursing homes and five or six times in hospital. There was a wide variation in the use of hospitals for short-term breaks. One person had eight stays during the study period in hospital and two others, five stays; most of the remainder had just one or two. The picture was more uniform in residential and nursing homes, with one person having five stays, one four stays and the remainder one or two stays. Average total cost of short-term breaks during the study period was £805 for people staying in homes, £3,726 for those staying in hospital.

Spreading the costs over the study period, the mean cost was estimated as £37 (median £29) per week in residential and nursing homes and £147 in hospital (median £129). Considering that so few people received short-term breaks in hospital (just nine), the contribution to the package cost was considerable when average total package costs are considered (£10 per week). This is one reason for the skewed distribution of health service costs of people cared for in the community discussed below. Residential home-based short-term breaks added just £3.50 per week to average package costs of the sample.

Lifetime costs of short-term care

Another approach to estimating the use and costs of short-term breaks is the lifetime use of the service. When information was included about use of short-term breaks before Time One, 30 people at some point had used either hospital (*n*=12) or residential (*n*=20) based short-term breaks, two of whom had used both; 12 of these had stayed only once, either as a one-off stay or as a trial admission prior to long-term care. Nobody currently using the service identified any short-term breaks more than 15 months before the Time One interview. Overall average number of stays since the older person started to receive short-term breaks was twice in residential and nursing homes and five times in hospital. In the study period, there were a few people who influenced the hospital pattern of use of short-term breaks. For example, one person had 13 stays in hospital prior to her death. The picture was again more consistent in the use of residential and nursing homes: two people had five stays, two three stays and the remainder one or two stays.

Average cost per stay recorded in residential or nursing homes was £480 (median value £430), and in hospital it was £1,278 (median value £1,600). Average length of stay was similar to the study period: 11 days in both venues, largely reflecting the balance between one and two-week stays. In total, people stayed an average of 52 days (median 16.5 days) in hospital and 21 days (median 17.5 days) in residential care. This translated into an average total lifetime cost per person receiving short-term breaks of £899 (median value £574) for people using residential and nursing homes and £5,859 (median value £1,887) for people using hospital. This excluded the final stay if it ended in death or permanent care.

Clearly, for those people still living in the community there may well be future short-term breaks. Although the numbers become very small, it is of interest to contrast the lifetime use of the service between those who have died or entered permanent care and those who are still living in the community. For those still in the community (nine people) who had short stays in residential or nursing homes, the level of consumption of service up to the Time Two interview was lower than those who had died or entered permanent care (*n*=11) (18 and 24 days, respectively). The picture was different among older people who had short-term breaks in hospital. The use of short-term breaks was about the same for those who died or entered permanent care (eight people staying 52 days on average), compared with those who remained in the community (four people, staying 52 days on average).

Package costs

Tables 8.2 and 8.3 show mean and median package costs respectively. Local authority purchased and provided and NHS packages are distinguished by area together with estimated accommodation costs of living in the community. Residential care costs are shown with estimates to cover additional service receipt and living expenses not covered by the establishment. This allows comparison of like with like in considering the total costs of care. Information about service receipt was sufficiently detailed to estimate package costs for 127 people: 120 for whom service costs were known and a further seven known not to be receiving any services.

Table 8.2: Mean weekly costs of packages of care

	Metropolitan borough (£)	London borough* (£)	County (£)	Total (£)
Costs of community services by local authority				
Local authority purchased services	47.56	118.32	75.87	70.49
NHS services	47.99	96.04	51.37	57.74
Accommodation costs and living expenses	193.33	161.75	185.92	185.01
Base (n)	(36)	(14)	(29)	(79)
Total package of community care	**279.66**	**376.11**	**313.15**	**309.05**
Costs of residential services by local authority				
Residential care	267.70	328.96	281.11	286.09
Additional services	13.39	16.45	14.06	14.30
Personal expenses	13.35	13.35	13.35	13.35
Base (n)	(25)	(12)	(11)	(48)
Total package of residential care	**294.72**	**358.76**	**308.52**	**313.75**
Total	**285.72**	**368.11**	**311.88**	**310.82**

*Including an allowance for higher costs in London, weekly costs would be: NHS services in London borough, £116.61; total package of community care in London borough, £396.68; total cost of residential care in London borough, £379.18; total cost of NHS services £61.39; total package of community care, £312.69; total cost of residential care in £313.00

Table 8.3: Median weekly costs of packages of care

	Metropolitan borough (£)	London borough* (£)	County (£)	Total (£)
Costs of community services by local authority				
Local authority purchased services	27.65	105.28	72.30	46.20
NHS services	2.46	22.75	6.68	3.62
Accommodation costs and living expenses	173.92	161.56	170.86	170.86
Base (n)	(36)	(14)	(29)	(79)
Total package of community care	**271.58**	**305.35**	**291.92**	**280.39**
Costs of residential services by local authority				
Residential care	278.80	327.89	246.00	298.55
Additional services	13.94	16.39	12.30	14.93
Personal expenses	13.35	13.35	13.35	13.35
Base (n)	(25)	(12)	(11)	(48)
Total package of residential care	**306.09**	**357.63**	**271.65**	**326.83**
Total	**275.30**	**346.81**	**286.16**	**292.31**

*Including an allowance for higher costs in London, weekly costs would be: total package of community care in London borough, £310.62; overall total 293.31. Other figures would remain unchanged.

Accommodation costs and living expenses for those people receiving community-based packages appear to be lower in the London borough. This reflects the living circumstances of the older people rather than costs of accommodation, which had been estimated to reflect the higher housing costs in London. In the London borough a lower proportion of older people lived in owner-occupied housing and a higher proportion in flats as opposed to whole houses.

Local authority purchased and provided service packages reflected the relative unit costs and prices of services in each area. Further analyses of the relationship between costs of local authority arranged packages over the study period and needs-related circumstances would allow a better understanding of cost variations between areas and between individuals.

Community health service costs exclude inpatient care, as the receipt of this service is not regarded as part of the package of care. (For the most part, inpatient stays were for planned operations.) Short-term breaks in hospital were included.

There was a considerable range in the costs associated with NHS service receipt. Using unit costs for day hospital and hospital based health services which reflect London costs, average costs of health service receipt were very similar to local authority purchased and provided community services in the metropolitan borough and the London borough. But the much lower median figure indicates that this was a function of relatively few very high-cost cases. Once residential based care is taken into consideration, however, local authority purchased or provided services dominate in all areas.

Including living expenses, the cost of care in the community for this client group appears similar to the cost of residential based care. The average picture conceals considerable variation in service package costs, however. Further analysis is needed to explore reasons behind variation in total costs of packages and to set these in the context of outcomes over the study period.

Conclusion

It has been possible to provide only a broad description of the methodology, resulting costs of services received and packages of care that people were receiving at the beginning of the study period. The study has provided an opportunity to explore the patterns and cost implications of short-term breaks receipt, an area where there is a lack of information about current practice. Overall package costs reflect the characteristics of the three local authorities in terms of unit costs of provision.

9

Conclusions

Key points

- This chapter draws together the key findings and main messages from the study.

- The framework for the evaluation was multidimensional. It offered evidence on community care for people with dementia in terms of patterns of service use, factors associated with entry to long-term care, the costs of community and long-term care services, the contribution of carers and the perspectives of carers and people with dementia.

- As people with dementia are major users of community and long-term care services, SSDs must ensure that their commissioning strategies are designed to address the specific needs of this client group.

- The experiences of carers showed continuities and contrasts with existing research, highlighting the need for services to develop in ways that take account of demographic and social change.

- The study offers new information on the views of people with moderate and severe dementia about community and long-term services.

"You've got to stamp your feet until you get answers.... I'm prepared to do the best I can for her [mother-in-law] but there are times when it's difficult and it puts a strain on family relationships.... If you [were to] ask for more help than we are getting at the moment, it would cost more than to put her in a home. But some say that's not true. [You get] conflicting information." (Mrs Richard, caring for her mother-in-law at Time Two)

Introduction

Across all groups of older people, research comparing service users with non-service users has suggested that increasing age, functional status and self-perceived health are the strongest predictors of service use (Bowling et al, 1993). Studies of people living in the community show that people with dementia use more services than older people without cognitive impairment, particularly in terms of those services that are arranged by SSDs (Cullen et al, 1993; Livingston et al, 1990; O'Connor et al, 1989b). People with cognitive impairment make up a large proportion of people needing long-term care or intensive community support (MRC CFAS and RIS, 1999). The implementation of the 1990 NHS and Community Care Act in April 1993 highlighted the need for information from studies that were able to document community care for people with dementia in the context of the new arrangements for funding, assessment and service provision.

Reasons for examining how SSDs arrange and provide services for people with dementia

There were a number of important reasons for undertaking a study examining how SSDs were arranging community care for people with dementia:

- While SSDs had the responsibility as 'lead agency' in assessing people's needs for community care, existing research had suggested that some traditional forms of service provision were not suited to meeting the needs of people with dementia and their carers.

- There was little information comparing people with dementia across the community and in long-term care settings post-April 1993, although SSD community care budgets covered both settings.

- One of the key aims of the community care changes was to provide better support for carers, and existing research had suggested that carers of people with dementia are at greater risk of psychological ill-health than other types of carer.

- There was a growing recognition of user views, yet the ability of people with dementia to offer their opinion on services was underestimated.

- The multiple needs of people with dementia provided a good testing ground for the effectiveness of working relationships between health, housing and SSDs.

- As SSDs improved their capacity to attach costs to services, more information on the costs of care for people with dementia was needed.

What did the study involve?

Information on people who had been referred to SSDs in three areas was collected over a four-month period from November 1994 to February 1995. Referral records from 14 social work teams were screened in order to identify people aged 65 and over who had gone on to receive an assessment and who had signs of cognitive impairment that were suggestive of dementia. Confirmation of suitability for inclusion in the study was made through interviews with their assessor, usually a social

worker. Once families had agreed to participate in the study, information was collected through a series of separate interviews with carers, proxy informants and people with dementia (Time One). They were reinterviewed approximately 11 months later (Time Two).

What happened to participants in the study?

At the time of referral, all but nine of the 141 study participants lived in the community. When the Time One interviews with the older people and carers or proxy informants took place, approximately six months after the referral and five months after the assessment, three fifths still lived at home. By Time Two, on average some 18 months after the referral, the proportion was less than a third. One in seven had died.

What implications does the study have for future research?

Research using assessors as informants

The period of time required in order to set up the study and recruit the sample was considerable. Other work has documented how front-line staff view increased paperwork and bureaucracy as a negative byproduct of the community care changes (Levin and Webb, 1997; Lewis and Glennerster, 1996; Petch et al, 1996). We were advised that asking practitioners to complete lengthy forms might reduce their willingness to participate in the research. However, when they were asked to take part in semi-structured interviews to confirm who was, and who was not, eligible for inclusion in the study, it was striking how many of the assessors went to considerable lengths to check records and supply details about their assessments. Interviews generally do take longer to complete than self-completion questionnaires but this method appeared to reduce the amount of data for which there were missing values. In addition, we were able to cross-check interview information against lists of referrals in order to quantify the number of people for whom we did not have information.

Research with service providers

Almost all the proxy informants were paid staff working in long-term care. We have drawn attention to the way in which some proxy informants felt that they lacked information about the person with dementia or were not involved in decision making. This should not just be seen as a research issue relating simply to the quality of the data. It has implications for the care that they were able to provide. Specific techniques for working with clients with dementia, such as life story books and reminiscence work, and the principles behind the person-centred care approach require that staff acquire knowledge about the life of the person with dementia.

The original purpose of the interviews with proxy informants was primarily to find out details of service receipt (see next section). However, what also emerged from the interviews was the differing approaches to caring for people with dementia and the differing levels of experience among the proxy informants. It highlighted how the perspectives of staff working with people with dementia in social care settings is an under-researched issue.

Research with carers

There is already a substantial literature of research on caring. The study confirmed how important it is to be able to examine caring from different perspectives – gender, household type, the kin relationship between the carer and the person cared for – and to compare people currently supporting someone living at home with people caring for someone in long-term care. Results from the study showed the importance of taking account of specific aspects of caring, such as giving high levels of personal care, or the impact of behavioural problems. However, the broader context of carers' social support, income and employment status must also be considered in research on caring. Here, a broader social science research approach appears to have advantages over those that consider caring simply in terms of the absence or presence of psychological ill-health. Future research could try to examine the interaction between the direct impact of caring (such as hours and type of care given) and its indirect impact (for instance, the long-term effects of caring on social networks) and factors independent of caring, such as life events.

Participating in research that offers no direct benefits demands high levels of commitment and altruism on the part of carers. Carers were included on the research advisory group, and they made valuable and useful suggestions about the content of interview schedules and how study findings related to their own experience.

Research with people with dementia

Over the last few years, there has been increasing recognition that people with dementia should be consulted about their experiences of service receipt. The study adds to the small but growing literature confirming that people with moderate and severe dementia can comment on the services they receive (Bamford, 1998; Levin et al, 1994; Mozley et al, 1999). Although some participants were unable to speak owing to the severity of their dementia, many more were able to offer an opinion. On the whole, they had more to say about services received on a daily basis, such as home care and day care, than about services that were used irregularly, such as short-stay care, or were one-off events, such as assessment.

Details of service receipt were confirmed before each interview (with the person with dementia) took place. This was useful when participants were unsure about or denied receiving a service. It also avoided causing potential distress by directly confronting people with memory deficits by asking, for instance, how often they attended day care.

Some people with dementia were not interviewed because their carer felt that questions designed to measure cognitive impairment might cause distress. This is an important issue. As public awareness of dementia increases, participants in research are increasingly aware of the purpose of questions designed to test short-term memory. It is possible that there will be an overall reduction in people's willingness to comply with screening instruments. At the same time, if no standardised measures are used, then it will not be possible to place their other responses within the context of their overall level of cognitive impairment. The Alzheimer's Society research programme, Quality Research in Dementia, will give carers and people with dementia a direct say in setting the research agenda and in the reporting of research results. It may contribute to producing a compromise to the dilemma of finding standardised measures that have good reliability and validity but do not cause distress and anxiety when administered.

What information does the study offer on the accessibility of SSD services?

Information on the agency making the referral showed that just under half of the referrals, including those for all older people, not just those identified as meeting the criteria for inclusion in the study, came from health sources. This emphasises the importance of strategies designed to improve partnerships between health and social services.

In addition to referrals from health sources, a high proportion of referrals came from families themselves. This is consistent with the results from other studies completed post-April 1993 (Edwards and Kenny, 1997) but contrasts with research completed prior to April 1993 which suggested that it was unusual for families to contact statutory services directly themselves (Sinclair et al, 1990). In this study, nearly a third of referrals had been made by families on behalf of the person with dementia. This should be seen as reflecting positively on the work that the study SSDs had undertaken in improving awareness of the help that they could offer through information leaflets and other local publicity.

Although three quarters of the people with dementia in the study had a carer who was able to make a referral on his or her behalf, some study participants did not have any family or friends. These people were often referred only when signs that the deterioration in their cognitive function had became overt, for example, if they began wandering at night or causing a disturbance.

What information does the study offer on identifying needs within the local population?

It has been suggested that SSDs need more sophisticated population needs assessments to help them identify at-risk groups (DoH Social Care Group, 1999). SSDs will derive useful information from comparing information on the demographic characteristics of their referral population with the characteristics of the local population as a whole. In particular, it will become more readily apparent when certain groups represented in the population living locally are under-represented in the referral population.

Overall, very few of the 1,258 referrals on which we collected information were for people from minority ethnic groups (Moriarty and Webb, 1995). Although the age structure of Britain's minority ethnic group population is slightly different from that of the white population, it is set to change. This means that SSDs can expect to see an increase in the number of referrals of older people from minority ethnic groups. There is an urgent need for a better infrastructure in order to meet the increasing needs of people with dementia from minority ethnic groups (Patel et al, 1998).

The age, gender, and social class of study participants and the proportion with access to a carer were similar to those found in representative samples of people with dementia derived from GP age–sex registers. However, a higher proportion of study participants had severe dementia and proportionally more lived alone. Our methods of sample selection meant that it is possible that some clients with dementia who met the criteria for inclusion in the study were excluded. However, the lack of information that is currently available on the prevalence of dementia among older SSD clients means that we have no way of knowing whether the study participants were similar to those found in other SSDs serving similar populations.

There is evidence that it is hard to extract information on the number of people with dementia using SSD services from SSD information systems (SSI, 1996), and this influenced the methods of sample selection that were available to us.

It is possible that public health departments within health authorities could be one source of useful advice for SSDs in terms of estimating the numbers of people with dementia that they might expect to see based on the age structure of their local population. Another solution to the problem in identifying people with dementia in local populations is through the development of case registers, shared jointly between health and social services (Cooper and Fearn, 1998).

What information does the study offer on estimating spending and service needs for the future?

Comparisons between the costs of community care and residential care

There is very little published information on the costs of care for people with dementia based on data collected since April 1993, except for the study completed by Livingston and colleagues (1997) on the costs of dementia care packages received by people living in the community. The costings completed by Dr Ann Netten, Angela Hallam and Jane Knight from the Personal Social Services Research Unit suggested that the costs of community care services in the study areas were similar to the costs of residential care.

The existence of the residential allowance can make it cheaper for SSDs to provide residential care than community services, although *Modernising social services* (Secretary of State for Health, 1998) has promised that it will be replaced by a fairer system. Most SSDs currently offer ceilings on the packages of community care services (Challis et al, 1998). The comparability of the costs of community services with costs of residential care should be viewed in the context that they did not enable substantial levels of community services to be purchased. At times of tightening SSD budgets, cost constraints could outweigh the preferences of client themselves.

We are not able to relate information on costs with outcomes in this book. This is an important requirement for work in the future. In particular, the evidence that ceilings for community care

packages are based largely on cost alone (Challis et al, 1998) highlights the need for more information on the levels of service receipt that would be required and at what cost in order to maintain people with different levels of cognitive impairment at home.

In this context, it is important to consider the positive results that were obtained through survival analyses. They suggested that people with home care and day care were more likely to remain at home. The study design does not allow causal explanations between service receipt and outcome to be offered. However, the analyses were able to control for severity of cognitive impairment, access to a carer, service receipt and the SSD in which participants lived. They are important in the light of concerns that the development of community services is being constrained because of the increasing numbers of existing clients in long-term care whom SSDs have a commitment to fund (Edwards and Kenny, 1997) and the pressures on budgets for older people's services from other areas of local authority expenditure, such as children's services or education.

It is also important that future work is able to look at the overall costs of dementia care within localities. Historically, both SSD and health provision for people with dementia has developed unevenly in different parts of the country. The study showed that the costs to the NHS of supporting study participants differed across the three SSDs. It is quite possible that these results are attributable to the methods of sample selection in that we have no way of knowing whether NHS services within the study areas were supporting large numbers of people with dementia who were not referred to the SSD during the period over which we collected referrals. However, the results serve to highlight the need for more information to help clarify where equitable health and social care provision is compromised by low levels of expenditure on dementia care, within both SSDs and health authorities.

Developing new forms of service provision

The identification of the costs associated with community and residential services in the study provides useful information about developing services in the future.

Short-stay care was estimated as being 10% more costly per week than a permanent place in long-term care. NHS short-stay care was identified as being particularly costly. At the same time, the numbers of SSDs who are reducing or contracting-out their residential provision means that the other mainstay of short-stay provision, the local authority home, is becoming more uncommon. The development of short-stay care in the voluntary and private sectors has been slow, yet many carers felt that small, homely environments offered a better alternative to NHS wards or large local authority homes.

Many carers find that offers of short-term care pose uncomfortable dilemmas. While they are adamant that for the sake of their own health they need to use the service, equally, they feel guilty if the person with dementia does not appear to have enjoyed his or her stay. In our study, short-term care was offered in very traditional ways. In this sense, there was less choice of provision than in the respite care study, where a small number of people had tried adult or family-based placement (Levin et al, 1994).

The *Carers' strategy* (HM Government, 1999) makes new funding available for services to support carers. While there is no doubt that in some circumstances short-term care should be provided in the NHS (for instance, distinctions between short stays and in-depth assessments can be blurred), there is the potential for health and social services to work together, using funds released from reducing short-stay care in NHS wards with new money from the *Carers strategy*, to develop alternative services that are more in accordance with the preferences of carers and people with dementia.

The study suggested that another area in which services might be developed was in providing intensive emergency support when people with dementia, or their carers, had a temporary need for increased help. At the time when data for the study were being collected, the only temporary additional help offered was through standard home care provision or short-stay care. Nationally, there are examples of schemes designed to provide this sort of assistance, but such provision has tended to remain

outside the mainstream. Joint investment plans, where health and social services work together on avoiding unnecessary admissions to care homes and hospitals, are one avenue through which these types of development might be considered.

Estimating future spending needs

The study suggested that, over time, the risk of entry to long-term care among participants increased. The average interval from referral to entry to long-term care among people with severe cognitive impairment was seven months; for people with mild cognitive impairment it was 13, and for people with moderate cognitive impairment it was 16.

It was also clear that there was considerable variation in the length of time for which participants used long-term care. At Time Two, over 80% (n=29) of the 35 people in residential care at Time One were still there; one person had been transferred to nursing care and five people had died. Of the 14 people living in nursing homes, six had died by Time Two and the remainder were still living there. The increase in the number of people in long-term care meant that the proportion of fully or partially local authority funded residents in long-term care had risen from 66% at Time One to 87% at Time Two.

While the study does provide some information on the use of estimating spending needs for the future, the need for better information on long-term service use remains. The study design did not take account of whether the referral represented participants' first contact with the SSD or whether they were existing users. Research looking at the use of services over a longer period would offer a clearer picture of the balance between community and long-term care service use by people with dementia. Given that so many SSD clients, not just people with dementia, use services over a number of years, it might also offer evidence on whether calculating the Standard Spending Assessment (SSA) annually is the most effective way of helping SSDs plan their spending on community care.

What information does the study offer on improving practice in assessment and care management?

Response times and involving carers

Over 80% of study participants had been assessed within one month of referral. It was clear that successful arrangements for notifying users and carers in advance of the date and time of the assessment were in place in all of the study SSDs, with around three quarters of the carers reporting that they had been given a precise date and time for the assessment. Of these, almost three quarters had been present for the assessment of the person for whom they cared.

Identifying health needs

Although the study was not designed to monitor the extent of unrecognised health needs in SSD populations, research that has done this suggests that high levels of unmet health needs can occur (Redmond et al, 1996). It has been suggested that depression, in particular, may be under-recognised in users of home care services (Banerjee and Macdonald, 1996; Banerjee et al, 1996) and in people living in residential care (Schneider et al, 1997b). The study findings were consistent with existing research on the extent of untreated depression in long-term care.

Although the NHS provided the largest single source of referrals, many study participants had been referred by family and friends, the general public and other social care agencies. It appeared that the social work teams received referrals for people with dementia who were not previously known to specialist health services. In this context, it is important that SSD assessments are able to identify potential unmet health needs in order that they can be brought to the attention of the person's GP.

On the basis of information provided by the assessors, it appeared that just under half of the assessments of study participants involved consultation with another professional. About a third of all the assessments resulted in a joint assessment at which the SSD assessor, other

professional(s) and the person with dementia all met together. It appeared that logistical considerations played a role in facilitating joint assessments, with hospital social workers being especially likely to have assessed jointly or consulted with another professional. The project 'Integrating social and health care: A comparative study of outcomes for older people and their carers' examines whether different approaches to collaboration, such as sharing the same workbase (co-location) between primary care and social care, result in improve outcomes for users (Levin and Iliffe, 1998).

Priorities for training

The development of a national training organisation (NTO) (Secretary of State for Health, 1998) provides an excellent opportunity for considering some of the priorities for training within the social care workforce. Social workers have been shown to have varying levels of knowledge about dementia (SSI, 1996), although it is an area in which many would like further training (Levin and Webb, 1997). Their access to appropriate training may be variable (Marshall, 1997).

Comments from carers and older people suggested that they valued the interpersonal and professional qualities of assessors. However, their experiences of assessments were very variable. The nature of the practice skills needed in order to work with people with dementia and their carers is an important issue. More work should be undertaken with practitioners on identifying key skills that they need.

Screening for cognitive impairment

The carers' comments suggested that some assessors had included questions designed to screen for cognitive impairment but that this practice was not universal. There is scope for SSDs to consider the feasibility of including short measures designed to screen for cognitive impairment in assessment proforma.

Identifying carers' needs

Three types of carer – co-resident carers, non-resident carers and former carers – were interviewed as part of this study. The evidence suggested that current co-resident carers were at greatest risk of psychological ill-health, that they were most affected by behavioural problems in the person for whom they cared, and that they had less social support than other carers. Most co-resident carers were the spouse of the person for whom they cared. Some carers had low incomes. These results are very consistent with those obtained in other research and highlight how assessors must be especially aware that carers of people with dementia are likely to have needs of their own. Assessors also need to increase carers' awareness of the full range of support available, including benefits advice and practical advice on caring for someone with dementia.

Using screening measures in practice settings

One of the problems in helping practitioners identify cognitive impairment or carers who are having difficulties is that instruments used in research are often too long and complicated for use in practice settings. Some may require pre-training. The NISW Noticeable Problems (Levin et al, 1989) is a six-item informant questionnaire that requires no pre-training, only that the informant be familiar with the older person. The Carers' Checklist (Hodgson et al, 1998) has been piloted extensively with carers and practitioners. Assessors may find that it is useful way of monitoring areas in which carers feel they are managing and areas in which they would like help.

However effective the screening instrument, there will always be problems in introducing routine measures where practitioners have no sense of ownership. Future research could try to identify whether consultation and discussion with practitioners results in more widespread use of standardised measures. It should also examine the degree to which practitioners find them useful in day-to-day practice.

Care management systems

The progressive nature of dementia means that the need for services is likely to be long-term and to increase over time. Sudden changes can also occur. There is a need for care management systems that are responsive to sudden changes as well as sensitive to gradual progressive deterioration. About two thirds of participants appeared to have had their care

reviewed between Times One and Two. However, sometimes services ceased when the person with dementia decided to stop using a service. It should not be assumed that the family will contact the SSD asking for alternative forms of assistance when this happens. Monitoring systems should be able to pick up when services cease in order to see whether an alternative form of care can be provided. The way in which information passed between people with dementia, carers, assessors and providers was variable, highlighting the need for effective systems for sharing information with all those who are involved in the care of the person with dementia.

The study was not designed to look at care management in detail. This means that we can only point to the contrast between the type of care management received by study participants, which accords with the administrative model most usually found within most SSDs (Challis et al, 1998), and the intensive models of care management designed to deal with people with complex long-term needs. Within the overall framework for assessing SSDs performance, there must be an acceptance that people with dementia may need a different type of service. For example, the process of assessing people with dementia is likely to be more expensive than assessing other types of client in view of the increased costs associated with consulting health, negotiating with more than one provider, and involving families. Extra time may be needed to help people with dementia reach a decision about whether or not to use a service. However, increased assessment costs can be justified if they result in more stable and effective packages of care. The low number of admissions to long-term care in the interval between the assessment and Time One suggested that assessments were an effective means of identifying where community care was feasible and where long-term care was required.

What information does the study offer on how well the needs of people with dementia were being met?

Community services

Results from the study suggested that changes to home care services had resulted in a service that was better able to meet the needs of carers and people with dementia. First, changes in the intensity of the service have made it more suitable for people who require frequent assistance, such as those with dementia. Home care was provided an average of seven times per week, spread over five days. The average amount of home care provided per week was five hours. While this represents a lower level of provision than that provided to people with dementia in a specialist care management service (Challis et al, 1997), it does show an improvement on levels of provision in studies completed prior to the community care changes (Levin et al, 1989).

Second, while neighbours might provide help with shopping, assistance with personal care is almost always provided by families (Parker and Lawton, 1994; Qureshi and Walker, 1989; Wenger, 1992). Assistance with personal care and meal preparation represents an improvement on traditional home care and meals services, which had been identified as not meeting the needs of people with dementia and their families (O'Connor et al, 1989b).

Day care remained the main way in which the leisure and social needs of people with dementia could be met. It was also most carers' main source of a regular break. However, not all people with dementia enjoy day care. Others have needs that are too great to be catered for in day centres with standard staffing levels. The failure to develop more home-based carer support within the study SSDs reflects the way in which too narrow a focus on assistance with personal care has prevented home care services from realising their full potential. It means that people with dementia who cannot or do not wish to attend day care are at risk of social exclusion.

Long-term care

The increased risk of entry to long-term care for people with dementia highlights how consideration must be given to making the process of moving into long-term care less distressing. While some people with dementia had made a successful transition, others spoke about their unhappiness at leaving their home. As was discussed in the section on screening, the finding that almost half of the people with dementia in long-term care were also suffering from a depressive illness suggests that more attention needs to be paid to the identification of depression among older people in this setting.

Supporting people with dementia who do not have carers

The inclusion of people with and without carers in the study highlighted the contrasts between the social networks of the two groups. Although three quarters of the people with dementia had a carer and two thirds saw other relatives regularly, only two fifths were reported to see friends. There was a group of people who had very little social contact with anyone other than staff working in home care, day care and long-term care. In some cases this was a continuation of their former life-style and a reflection of their own preference for privacy and solitude. In others it was not, as their answers to the questions on the BAS showed. There is an opportunity to develop befriending and advocacy schemes to support people with dementia who may not have any other family and friends.

What information does the study offer on how well the needs of carers are being met?

Information needs

The extent to which carers' information needs had been met was very variable. On the one hand, many carers reported that they had contacted the SSD of their own volition and that they knew who to contact if they wanted further help. Even so, many explained that, like Mrs Richards whose words opened this chapter, their knowledge had been hard won. On the other hand, many carers had been caring for several years prior to the referral without any support from statutory services. Their level of knowledge about potential sources of advice and the range of available services was quite poor. This remains very disappointing in view of the extensive research literature that already exists on carers' needs for more information.

Types of information needed

The carers' comments suggested that three sorts of information were required. First was information on diagnosis and prognosis. Here, their knowledge ranged from those who were familiar with the latest medical advances to those who said that no one had told them what was wrong with their relative. Old age psychiatry services and GPs should regularly review their strategies for making information available to carers.

Second, they needed information on the full range of services, in particular the possibility of home-based carer support, short-stay care and carers' groups. About a fifth of the carers who were re-interviewed had heard of the 1995 Carers (Recognition and Services) Act. None of them reported that they had asked for an assessment.

Finally, there was the potential for improving carers' familiarity with local and national voluntary organisations. The Alzheimer's Society, Counsel and Care, the Relatives' and Residents' Association and the Carers National Association all run helplines and provide information leaflets which could be particularly useful to people with dementia and their families. Carers in the study appeared to have been very reliant on the media for information about these organisations.

Social support

The lack of a confiding relationship may be associated with carer stress (Livingston et al, 1996). In this study, spouse carers whose children did not live locally tended to have fewer people to whom they could turn for support. Although many social workers appeared to be supporting those who were experiencing difficulties with their caring role, there were carers who wanted more support from professionals, in particular to have someone with whom to discuss how they were feeling. Many

social work practitioners feel that one consequence of the community care changes has been less opportunity for direct work with clients and their families (Levin and Webb, 1997). Current models of care management seem to neglect the role that social workers and CPNs had traditionally played in supporting people for whom they were the only source of social support.

Supporting former carers

There were signs that some residential and nursing homes in the study SSDs had facilitated the involvement of former carers in giving direct care. Some former carers said that they would contact the staff in long-term care, rather than the assessor or anyone else in the SSD, if they wanted to discuss the care of the person with dementia.

Nevertheless, some former carers, particularly spouses, had problems in visiting the person with dementia as often as they would have wished. Efforts should be made through volunteer driver or taxicard schemes to help former carers.

Some former carers reported financial problems following the loss of benefits or a reduction in their pension once the person they cared for was admitted to long-term care. When a period of caring ceases, because of either death or entry to long-term care, former carers should be helped with benefits advice.

Demographic and social change

Many carers under retirement age were in full or part-time paid employment. This reflected women's increasing participation in the labour force. At the same time, men under retirement age who were not in paid employment reported that they had started to care once they had given up paid employment for health reasons. While some carers lived within a short distance of the person for whom they cared, others had substantial journeys. Increased geographical mobility means that this is likely to become more common in the future. It is likely to place increased demands on home care to provide more services during the evenings and overnight.

Discussion

The study suggested that there were areas in which community care services within the study SSDs have resulted in some positive changes. Assessments seemed to have resulted in some successful and stable packages of community care services. However, over a quarter of the assessments resulted in offers of residential or nursing care, reflecting the way in which assessors are often dealing with people already at risk of entry to long-term care. There was strong evidence that long-term care was offered only to people with the highest levels of functional and cognitive disability.

The research supported the importance of collecting information on the severity of cognitive impairment at assessment. This was highlighted by the differential rate of entry to long-term care among study participants, in which those who were most severely cognitively impaired moved into long-term care within a short space of time after their referral.

At the same time, the degree to which users and carers were able to exercise choice was variable. Although the results suggested that greater consultation with carers took place in the process of assessment and arranging services, the amount of feedback they received remained patchy. It suggested that more attention should be given to the way in which information is passed on, especially as this is an area where the resource implications are comparatively small. The hours and days of the week over which home care was provided was more intensive than in the past and the assistance with personal care and meals was appreciated. However, day care and short-term care were still delivered in very traditional ways, suggesting that there were opportunities both to develop these services more flexibly and also to find alternative types of provision. Further work is needed to identify the extent to which the multiple and wide ranging requirements of older people with dementia and their carers are reflected in standard assessment and care management procedures.

The study showed that the referral of an older person with dementia to their local SSD represented the start of a relatively long-term relationship in which high-quality services could make a substantial difference to the way in which they and their carers were supported. In an inclusive society, social policy and welfare provision for this group of service users must better reflect their needs and wishes. The study demonstrated that it was possible to document the views of people with dementia, and we must conclude with a request from one of the study participants. At the beginning of the interview, Mrs Johns was told that the research was funded by the Department of Health. At the end, she turned to the interviewer and laughed:

> *"Now that I've answered all these questions for the government, do you think they'll do anything to give me more pension!"*

As the ability of people with dementia to give their views on services is becoming more widely accepted, the next challenge will be to ensure that future service provision will be comprehensive enough in its ability to meet their wide-ranging needs and varied enough to suit their diverse preferences.

References

ADSS (Association of Directors of Social Services) (1994) *Towards community care: ADSS review of the first year*, ADSS.

Akehurst, R., Hutton, J. and Dixon, R. (1991) *Review of higher costs of health care provision in inner London and a consideration of implications for competitiveness: Final report*, York: York Health Economics Consortium, University of York.

Allen, C. and Beecham, J. (1993) 'Costing services: ideals and reality', in A. Netten and J. Beecham (eds) *Costing community care: Theory and practice*, Aldershot: Ashgate.

Allen N. and Burns, A. (1995) 'The noncognitive features of dementia', *Reviews in Clinical Gerontology*, vol 5, pp 57-75.

Allen, N., Ames, D., Ashby, D., Bennetts, K., Tuckwell, V. and West, C. (1994) 'A brief sensitive screening instrument for depression in late life', *Age and Ageing*, vol 23, pp 213-18.

Amar, K. and Wilcock, G. (1996) 'Vascular dementia', *BMJ*, vol 312, pp 227-31.

American Psychiatric Association (1994) *Diagnostic and statistical manual of mental disorders*, 4th edn, Washington, DC: American Psychiatric Association.

Arber, S. and Ginn, J. (1991) *Gender and later life*, London: Sage Publications.

Arber, S. and Ginn, J. (1992) 'Class and caring: a forgotten dimension', *Sociology*, vol 26, pp 619-34.

Ashby, D., West, C. and Ames, D. (1989) 'The ordered logistic regression model in psychiatry: rising prevalence of dementia in old people's homes', *Statistics in Medicine*, vol 8, pp 1317-26.

Askham, J. and Thompson, C. (1990) *Dementia and home care: A research report on a home care scheme for dementia sufferers*, Mitcham: Age Concern.

Audit Commission (1986) *Making a reality of community care*, London: Audit Commission.

Audit Commission (1993) *Taking care*, Bulletin, London: Audit Commission.

Audit Commission (1997) *The coming of age: Improving care services for older people*, London: Audit Commission.

Audit Commission (1999) *The price is right? Charges for council services (national report)*, London: Audit Commission.

Bamford, C. (1998) 'Consulting older people with dementia', *Cash and Care*, Newsletter of the Social Policy and Research Unit, vol 22, p 2.

Banerjee, S. (1993) 'Prevalence and recognition rates of psychiatric disorder in the elderly clients of a community care service', *International Journal of Geriatric Psychiatry*, vol 8, pp 125-31.

Banerjee, S. and Macdonald, A. (1996) 'Mental disorder in an elderly home care population: associations with health and social services use', *British Journal of Psychiatry*, vol 168, pp 750-6.

Banerjee, S., Shamash, K., Macdonald, A. and Mann, A. (1996) 'Randomised controlled trial of effect of intervention by psychogeriatric team on depression in frail elderly people at home', *BMJ*, vol 313, pp 1058-60.

Baragwanath, A. (1997) 'Bounce and balance: a team approach to risk management for people with dementia living at home', in M. Marshall (ed) *State of the art in dementia care*, London: Centre for Policy on Ageing, pp 102-6.

Barer, B.M. and Johnson, C.L. (1990) 'A critique of the caregiving literature', *The Gerontologist*, vol 30, pp 26-30.

Barnes, C. (1996) 'Where is "IT" at in UK social services and social work departments?', *New Technology in the Human Services*, vol 9, pp 12-17.

Bartlett, E. (1996) *Crisis care for people with dementia: A study of options for the Salisbury area*, Salisbury: Alzheimer's Disease Society.

Bebbington, A., Brown, P., Darton, R. and Netten, A. (1996) *Survey of admissions to residential and nursing homes for elderly people*, Discussion Paper 1222, Canterbury: Personal Social Services Research Unit.

Bennett, N., Jarvis, L., Rowland, O., Singleton, N. and Hasleden, L. (1996) *Living in Britain: Results from the 1994 General Household Survey*, London: HMSO.

Bond, J., Brookes, P., Carstairs, V. and Giles, L. (1980) 'The reliability of a survey psychiatric assessment schedule for the elderly', *British Journal of Psychiatry*, vol 137, pp 148-59.

Boneham, M., Williams, K., Copeland, J., McKibbin, P., Wilson, K., Scott, A. and Saunders, P. (1997) 'Elderly people from ethnic minorities in Liverpool: mental illness, unmet need, and barriers to service use', *Health and Social Care in the Community*, vol 5, pp 173-80.

Bourgeois, M.S., Schulz, R. and Burgo, L. (1996) 'Interviews for caregivers of patients with Alzheimer's Disease: a review and analysis of content, process and outcomes', *International Journal of Aging and Human Development*, vol 43, pp 35-92.

Bowling, A., Farquar, M. and Grundy, E. (1993) 'Who are the consistently high users of health and social services? A follow up study two and a half years later of people aged 85 at baseline', *Health and Social Care in the Community*, vol 1, pp 187-277.

Bowling, A., Farquar, M., Grundy, E. and Formby, J. (1992) *Psychiatric morbidity among people aged 85+: A follow-up study at two and a half years: Associations with changes in psychiatric morbidity*, Working Paper no 1, London: Institute of Gerontology.

Brodaty, H. and Gresham, M. (1992) 'Prescribing residential respite care for dementia: effects, side-effects, indications and dosage', *International Journal of Geriatric Psychiatry*, vol 7, pp 357-62.

Brown, G. (1974) 'Meaning, measurement and stress of life events', in B.S. Dohrenwend and B.P. Dohrenwend (eds) *Stressful life events, their nature and effects*, New York, NY: John Wiley.

Brown, P., Challis, D. and von Abendorff, R. (1996) 'The work of a community mental health team for the elderly: referrals, caseloads, contact history and outcomes', *International Journal of Geriatric Psychiatry*, vol 11, pp 29-39.

Buck, D., Gregson, B., Bamford, C., McNamee, P., Farrow, G., Bond, J. and Wright, K. (1997) 'Psychological distress among informal supporters of frail older people at home and in institutions', *International Journal of Geriatric Psychiatry*, vol 12, pp 737-44.

Burholt, V., Wenger, G. and Scott, A. (1997) 'Dementia, disability and contact with formal services: a comparison of dementia sufferers and non-sufferers in rural and urban settings', *Health and Social Care in the Community*, vol 5, pp 384-97.

Burns, A. (1996) 'Psychiatric symptoms and behavioural disturbances in dementia: a review of therapy', *International Psychogeriatrics*, vol 8 (Supplement 2), pp 201-7.

Butt, J. and Mirza, K. (1996) *Black care and black communities*, London: HMSO.

Caldock, K. (1992a) *The management of community care for elderly people after the White Paper*, Bangor: Centre for Social Policy Research and Development.

Caldock, K. (1992b) *The new assessment: Moving towards holism or new roads to fragmentation?*, Bangor: Centre for Social Policy Research and Development.

Caldock, K. (1992c) *Use of assessment tools and documentaion in community care: Observing and analysing practice*, Bangor: Centre for Social Policy Research and Development.

Carers (Recognition & Services) Act 1995, London: HMSO.

Carr, J. (1992) *Tayside Dementia Services Planning Survey*, Stirling: Dementia Services Development Centre.

Challis, D. (1992) 'Providing alternatives to long stay hospital care for frail elderly patients: is it cost effective?', *International Journal of Geriatric Psychiatry*, vol 7, pp 773-81.

Challis, D. (1994) *Implementing caring for people, care management: Factors influencing its development in the implementation of community care*, London: DoH.

Challis, D. and Darton, R. (1990) 'Evaluation research and experiment in social gerontology', in S. Peace (ed) *Researching social gerontology*, London: Sage Publications.

Challis, D., Carpenter, I. and Traske, K. (1996) *Assessment in continuing care homes*, Canterbury: Personal Social Services Research Unit.

Challis, D., von Abendorff, R., Brown, P. and Chesterman, J. (1997) 'Care management and dementia: an evaluation of the Lewisham intensive case management scheme', in S. Hunter (ed) *Dementia: Challenges and new directions*, London: Jessica Kingsley, pp 139-64.

Challis, D., Chessum, R., Chesterman, J., Luckett, R. and Woods, B. (1987) 'Community care for the frail elderly: an urban experiment', *British Journal of Social Work*, vol 18 (supplement), pp 13-42.

Challis, D., Darton, R., Hughes, J., Stewart, K. and Weiner, K. (1998) *Care management study: Report on national data*, London: DoH Social Care Group.

Challis, D., Darton, R., Johnson, L., Stone, M. and Traske, K. (1995) *Care management and health care of older people*, Aldershot: Ashgate.

Charlton, J., Patrick, D. and Peach, H. (1983) 'Use of multivariate measures of disability in health surveys', *Journal of Epidemiology and Community Health*, vol 37, pp 296-304.

CIPFA (Chartered Institute of Public Finance and Accountancy) (1992) *Housing Revenue Account Statistics (HRA), 1992-93*, London: CIPFA Statistical Information Service.

Clarke, C., Heyman, R., Pearson, P. and Watson, D. (1993) 'Formal carers: attitudes to working with the dementing elderly and their informal carers', *Health and Social Care*, vol 1, pp 227-38.

Cohen, J. and Fisher, M. (1987) 'Recognition of mental health problems by doctors and social workers', *Practice*, vol 3, pp 225-40.

Coles, R.J., Von Abendorff, R. and Herzberg, J.L. (1991) 'The impact of a new community mental health team on an inner city psychogeriatric service', *International Journal of Geriatric Psychiatry*, vol 6, no 1, pp 31-9.

Cooper, B. and Fearn, R. (1998) 'Dementia care needs in an area population: case register data and morbidity survey estimates', *International Journal of Geriatric Psychiatry*, vol 13, pp 550-5.

Copeland, J., Kelleher, M, Kellett, J., Gourlay, A, Gurland, B., Fleiss, J. and Sharpe, L. (1976) 'A semi-structured clinical interview for the assessment and diagnosis of mental state in the elderly: the Geriatric Mental State Schedule 1, Development and reliability', *Psychological Medicine*, vol 6, pp 439-49.

Cullen, M., Blizard, R., Livingston, G. and Mann, A. (1993) 'The Gospel Oak project 1987-1990: provision and use of community services', *Health Trends*, vol 25, pp 142-6.

Cumella, S., Mesurier, N. and Tomlin, H. (1996) *Social work in practice: An evaluation of the care management received by elderly people from social workers based in GP practices in South Worcestershire*, Worcester: Martley Press.

Dalley, G. (1988) *Ideologies of caring*, Basingstoke: Macmillan Education.

Davies, B. (1987) 'Equity and efficiency in community care: supply and financing in an age of fiscal austerity', *Ageing and Society*, vol 7, pp 161 74.

Davies, B. and Challis, D. (1986) *Matching resources to needs in community care: An evaluated demonstration of a long term care model*, Aldershot: Gower.

Davies, B. and Fernandez, J. with Nomer, B. (in press) *Needs, services, productivities, and efficiencies: Implications for policy*, Aldershot: Ashgate.

Davies, B., Bebbington, A. and Charnley, H. with Baines, B., Ferlie, E., Hughes, M. and Twigg, J. (1990) *Resources, needs and outcomes in community based care*, Aldershot: Gower.

Davis, A., Ellis, K. and Rummery, K. (1998) *Access to assessment: Perspectives of practitioners, disabled people and carers*, Bristol: The Policy Press.

Declaration of Helsinki (1964) Adopted by the 18th World Medical Assembly, Helsinki, Finland, 1964. Amended by the 29th World Medical Assembly, Tokyo, Japan, October 1975 and the 35th World Medical Assembly, Venice, Italy, October 1983.

DHSS (Department of Health and Social Security) (1981) *Report of a study on community care*, London: DHSS.

DoE (Department of the Environment) (1994) *Housing and Construction Statistics GB, 1983-93*, London: HMSO.

DoH (Department of Health) (1988) *Community care: An agenda for action*, London: HMSO.

DoH (1990) *Caring for people: Community care in the next decade and beyond, Policy Guidance*, London: HMSO.

DoH (1994) *Inspection of assessment and care management arrangements in social services departments: Second overview report*, London: DoH.

DoH (1997) *A handbook on the mental health of older people*, London: DoH.

DoH (1999) 'A new approach to social services performance: consultation responses and confirmation of performance indicators', Local Authority Circular (99) 27.

DoH Social Care Group (1999) *Meeting the challenge: Improving management information for the effective commissioning of social care services for older people, Management Summary*, London: DHSS.

Dunning, A. (1997) 'Advocacy and older people with dementia', in M. Marshall (ed) *Dementia: State of the art*, London: Centre for Policy on Ageing, pp 95-101.

Eagles, J., Craig, A., Rawlinson, F., Restall, D., Beattie, J. and Besson, J. (1987) 'The psychological well-being of supporters of the demented elderly', *British Journal of Psychiatry*, vol 150, pp 293-8.

ECCEP Team (1998) *ECCEP Bulletin*, Canterbury: Personal Social Services Research Unit.

Edwards, A. (1996) 'Is care managment being implemented?', *Community Care Management and Planning*, vol 4, pp 121-8.

Edwards, P. and Kenny, D. (1997) *Community care trends 1997*, London: Local Government Management Board.

Ely, M., Brayne, C., Huppert, F., O'Connor, D. and Pollitt, P. (1997) 'Cognitive impairment: a challenge for community care. A comparison of the domiciliary service receipt of cognitively impaired and equally dependent physically impaired elderly women', *Age and Ageing*, vol 26, pp 301-8.

Finch, J. and Groves, D. (eds) (1983) *A labour of love: Women, work and caring*, London: Routledge.

Fisher, M. (1990a) 'Care management and social work: clients with dementia', *Practice*, vol 4, pp 229-41.

Fisher, M. (1990b) 'Care management and social work: working with carers', *Practice*, vol 4, pp 242-52.

Fisher, M. (1994) 'Man-made care: community care and older male carers', *British Journal of Social Work*, vol 24, pp 659-80.

Fisher, M. (1998) 'The role of service users in problem formulation and technical aspects of social research', Paper presented at the seminar 'Formulating Research Problems in Practitioner-Researcher Partnerships', York.

Folstein, M., Folstein, S. and McHugh, P. (1975) '"Mini-Mental State" a practical method for grading the cognitive state of patients for the clinician', *Journal of Psychiatric Research*, vol 12, pp 189-98.

George, L.K. and Gwyther, L.P. (1986) 'Caregiver well-being: a multi-dimensional examination of family caregivers of demented adults', *The Gerontologist*, vol 26, pp 253-9.

Gilleard, C. (1992) 'Care services for the elderly mentally infirm', in G. Jones and B. Miesen (eds) *Care-giving in dementia*, London: Routledge.

Gilleard, C., Belford, H., Gilleard, E., Whittick, J. and Gledhill, K. (1984) 'Emotional distress amongst the supporters of the elderly mentally infirm', *British Journal of Psychiatry*, vol 145, pp 172-7.

Ginn, J. and Arber, S. (1996) 'Patterns of employment, gender and pensions: the effect of work history on older women's non-state pensions', *Work, Employment and Society*, vol 10, pp 469-90.

Goldberg, D. and Williams, P. (1988) *A user's guide to the general health questionnaire*, Windsor: NFER-Nelson Publishing Company.

Goldberg, E. and Warburton, R. (1979) *Ends and means in social work*, London: George Allen & Unwin.

Golden, R., Teresi, J. and Gurland, B. (1984) 'Development of indicator scales for the Comprehensive Assessment and Referral Evaluation (CARE) Interview Schedule', *Journal of Gerontology*, vol 39, pp 138-46.

Goldsmith, M. (1996) *Hearing the voice of people with dementia: Opportunities and obstacles*, London: Jessica Kingsley.

Goodacre, H. and Smith, R. (1997) 'The rights of patients in research', *BMJ*, vol 310, pp 1277-80.

Gordon, D., Spicker, P., Ballinger, B., Gillies, B., McWilliam, N., Mutch, W. and Seed, P. (1997) 'Identifying older people with dementia: the effectiveness of a multiservice census', *International Journal of Geriatric Psychiatry*, vol 12, pp 636-41.

Graham, C., Ballard, C. and Sham, P. (1997) 'Carers' knowledge of dementia and their expressed concerns', *International Journal of Geriatric Psychiatry*, vol 12, pp 470-3.

Graham, N. and Waldron, G. (1983) 'Medical and psychiatric characteristics of elderly persons', in E. Levin, I. Sinclair and P. Gorbach (eds) *The supporters of confused elderly persons at home, Vol 3, Appendices*, London: NISW Research Unit.

Grant, G. and Nolan, M. (1993) 'Informal carers: sources and concomitants of satisfaction', *Health and Social Care in the Community*, vol 1, pp 147-59.

Gray, A. and Fenn, P. (1993) 'Alzheimer's disease: the burden of the illness in England', *Health Trends*, vol 25, pp 31-7.

Green, H. (1988) *Informal carers*, OPCS Series GHS, No 15, Supplement A, London: HMSO.

Greene, J., Smith, R., Gardiner, M. and Timbury, G. (1982) 'Measuring behavioural disturbance of elderly demented patients in the community and its effects on relatives: a factor analytic study', *Age and Ageing*, vol 11, pp 121-6.

Gurland, B., Cross, P., Defiguerido, J., Shannon, M., Mann, A.H. and Jenkins, R. (1979) 'A cross-national comparison of the institutionalized elderly in the cities of New York and London', *Psychological Medicine*, vol 9, pp 781-8.

Halifax Building Society (1996) *House price index*, London: Halifax Building Society.

Harwood, D., Hope, T. and Jacoby, R. (1997) 'Cognitive impairment in medical inpatients, II: Do physicians miss cognitive impairment?', *Age and Ageing*, vol 26, pp 37-9.

Hatfield, B., Huxley, P., Mohamad, H., Mawer, J. and Ruffley, P. (1994) 'Supporting older people with dementia: the service needs of informal carers', *Social Services Research*, vol 4, pp 10-11.

Henwood, M. (1992) *Through a glass darkly: Community care and elderly people*, London: King's Fund Institute.

Her Majesty's Government (1999) *Caring about carers: A national strategy*, London: HMSO.

Higginson, I., Jeffries, P. and Hodgson, C. (1997) 'Outcome measures for routine use in dementia services: some practical considerations', *Quality in Health Care*, vol 6, pp 120-4.

Hinrichsen, G. and Niederehe, G. (1994) 'Dementia management strategies and adjustment of family members of older patients', *The Gerontologist*, vol 34, pp 95-102.

Hodgson, C., Higginson, I. and Jeffreys, P. (1998) *Carers' checklist: An outcome measure for people with dementia and their carers*, London: Mental Health Foundation.

Hofman, A., Rocca, W., Brayne, C., Breteler, M., Clarke, M., Cooper, B., Copeland, J., Dartigues, J., Droux, A., Hagnell, O., Heeren, T., Engedal, K., Jonker, C., Lindesay, J., Lobo, A., Mann, A., Mölsa, P., Morgan, K., O'Connor, D., Sulkava, R., Kay, D. and Amaducci, L. (1991) 'The prevalence of dementia in Europe: a collaborative study of 1980-1990 findings', *International Journal of Epidemiology*, vol 20, pp 736-48.

Hofman, A., Ott, A., Breteler, M.M.B., Botts, M.L., Slooter, A.J.C., Harskamp, F.v., Duijn, C.N.v., Broeckhoven, C.V. and Grobbee, D.E. (1997) 'Atherosclerosis, apolipoprotein E, and prevalence of dementia and Alzheimer's disease in the Rotterdam Study', *Lancet*, vol 349, pp 151-4.

Hope, T. and Patel, V. (1993) 'Assessment of behavioural phenomena in dementia', in A. Burns (ed) *Ageing and dementia: A methodological approach*, Sevenoaks, Kent: Edward Arnold, pp 221-36.

Hope, T., Keene, J., Gedling, K., Fairburn, C.G. and Jacoby, R. (1998). 'Predictors of institutionalization for people with dementia living at home with a carer', *International Journal of Geriatric Psychiatry*, vol 13, pp 682-90.

Hughes, B. (1993) 'A model for the comprehensive assessment of older people and their carers', *British Journal of Social Work*, vol 23, pp 345-64.

Hughes, B. (1995) *Older people and community care: Critical theory and practice*, Buckingham: Open University Press.

Hunter, S., Brace, S., and Buckley, G. (1993) 'The inter-disciplinary assessment of older people at entry to long term institutional care: lessons for the new community care arrangements', *Research, Policy and Planning*, vol 11, no 1/2, pp 2-9.

Iliffe, S., Mitchley, S., Gould, M. and Haines, A. (1994) 'Evaluation of the use of brief screening instruments for dementia, depression and problem drinking among elderly people in general practice', *British Journal of General Practice*, vol 44, pp 503-7.

Kavanagh, S. and Knapp, M. (1999) 'Cognitive disability and direct care costs for elderly people', *British Journal of Psychiatry*, vol 174, pp 539-46.

Keady, J. (1996) 'The experience of dementia: a review of the literature and implications for nursing practice', *Journal of Clinical Nursing*, vol 5, pp 275-88.

Kitwood, T. (1997) *Dementia reconsidered: The person comes first*, Buckingham: Open University Press.

Kitwood, T. and Bredin, K. (1992) 'Towards a theory of dementia care: personhood and well-being', *Ageing and Society*, vol 12, pp 269-70.

Knapp, M. (1993) 'Principles of applied cost research', in A. Netten and J. Beecham (eds) *Costing community care: Theory and practice*, Aldershot: Ashgate.

Knapp, M., Beecham, J. and Allen, C. (1989) *The methodology for costing community and hospital services used by clients of the care in the community demonstration programme*, Discussion Paper 647, Canterbury: Personal Social Services Research Unit.

Knapp, M., Wilkinson, D. and Wrigglesworth, R. (1998) 'The economic consequences of Alzheimer's disease in the context of new drug developments', *International Journal of Geriatric Psychiatry*, vol 13, pp 531-3.

Knight, B. (1996) *Representational advocacy in action*, Gateshead: Darlington CAB, Derwentside CAB and National Association of Citizens Advice Bureaux.

Knopman, D.S., Kitto, J., Deinard, S. and Heiring, J. (1988) 'Longitudinal study of death and institutionalization in patients with primary degenerative dementia', *Journal of the Americal Geriatrics Society*, vol 36, pp 108-12.

Leek, S. and Fletcher, C. (1996) *Home care services for people with dementia*, Wolverhampton: University of Wolverhampton Educational Research Unit.

Levin, E. (1997) 'Carers: problems, strains and services', in R. Jacoby and C. Oppenheimer (eds) *Psychiatry in the elderly*, 2nd edn, Oxford: Oxford University Press.

Levin, E. and Iliffe, S. (1998) 'Integrating social and health care: a comparative study of outcomes for older people and their carers', OSCA Project Summary Progress Report.

Levin, E. and Moriarty, J. (1996) 'Evaluating respite services', in R. Bland (ed) *Developing services for older people and their families*, London: Jessica Kingsley, pp 129-43.

Levin, E. and Webb, S. (1997) *Social work and community care: The changing roles and tasks*, London: NISW Research Unit.

Levin, E., Moriarty, J. and Gorbach, P. (1994) *Better for the break*, London: HMSO.

Levin, E., Sinclair, I. and Gorbach, P. (1989) *Families, services and confusion in old age*, Aldershot: Avebury.

Levin, E., Webb, S. and Netten, A. (1997) 'Assessing need, use of time and social work costs', in E. Levin and S. Webb, *Social work and community care: The changing roles and tasks*, London: NISW Research Unit.

Lewis, J. with Bernstock, P., Bovell, V. and Wookey, F. (1997) 'Implementing care management: issues in relation to the new community care', *British Journal of Social Work*, vol 27, pp 5-24.

Lewis, J. and Glennerster, H. (1996) *Implementing the new community care*, Buckingham: Open University Press.

Lewis, J. and Meredith, B. (1988) *Daughters who care: Daughters caring for mothers at home*, London: Routledge.

Lindow, V. (1999) 'Users' perspectives', in S. Balloch, J. Butt, M. Fisher and V. Lindow (eds) *Rights, needs, and the user perspective: A review of the National Health Service and Community Care Act 1990*, London: NISW and the Joseph Rowntree Foundation, pp 24-36.

Livingston, G., Manela, M. and Katona, C. (1996) 'Depression and other psychiatric morbidity in carers of elderly people living at home', *BMJ*, vol 312, pp 153-6.

Livingston, G., Manela, M. and Katona, C. (1997) 'Cost of community care for older people', *British Journal of Psychiatry*, vol 171, pp 56-69.

Livingston, G., Thomas, A., Graham, N., Blizard, B. and Mann, A. (1990) 'The Gospel Oak Project: the use of health and social services by dependent elderly people in the community', *Health Trends*, vol 22, pp 70-3.

Lloyd, M., Webb, S. and Singh, S. (1995) *General practitioners and the community care reforms*, London: Department of General Practice and Primary Care, Royal Free Hospital School of Medicine.

Local Authority Circular LAC (99) 27 (1999) *A new approach to social services performance: Consultation responses and confirmation of performance indicators*, London: DoH.

McCafferty, P. (1994) *Living independently: A study of the housing needs of elderly and disabled people*, Housing Research Report, DoE, London: HMSO.

Macdonald, A., Mann, A., Jenkins, R., Richard, L., Godlove, C. and Rodwell, G. (1982) 'An attempt to determine the impact of four types of care upon the elderly by the study of matched groups', *Psychological Medicine*, vol 12, pp 193-200.

MacDonald, C. (1999) *Support at home: Views of older people on their needs and access to services*, Edinburgh: The Stationery Office.

MacDonald, L., Higgs, P., MacDonald, J., Godfrey, E. and Ward, M. (1996) 'Carers' reflections on nursing home and NHS long-stay care for elderly patients', *Health and Social Care in the Community*, vol 4, no 5, pp 264-70.

McLaughlin, E. and Ritchie, J. (1994) 'Legacies of caring: the experiences and circumstances of ex-carers', *Health and Social Care*, vol 2, pp 241-53.

Maguire, C., Kirby, M., Coen, R., Coakley, D., Lawlor, B. and O'Neill, D. (1996) 'Family members' attitudes toward telling the patient with Alzheimer's disease their diagnosis', *BMJ*, vol 313, pp 529-30.

Mann, A., Graham, N. and Ashby, D. (1984) 'Psychiatric illness in residential homes for the elderly: a survey in one London borough', *Age and Ageing*, vol 13, pp 257-65

Mann, A., Ames, D., Graham, N., Weyerer, S., Eichhorn, S., Platz, S., Snowdon, J., Hughes, F. and Ticehurst, S. (1989) 'The reliability of the Brief Assessment Schedule', *International Journal of Geriatric Psychiatry*, vol 4, pp 221-5.

Manthorpe, J. (1994) 'The family and informal care', in N. Malin (ed) *Implementing community care*, Buckingham: Open University Press.

Marshall, M. (1997) 'Working with people with dementia', *Clinician*, vol 15, pp 38-44.

Meethan, K. and Thompson, C. (1993) *In their own homes: Incorporating carers' and users' views in care management*, York: Social Policy Research Unit.

Melzer, D., Ely, M. and Brayne, C. (1997) 'Cognitive impairment in elderly people: population based estimate of the future in England, Scotland, and Wales', *BMJ*, vol 315, p 462.

Melzer, D., Hopkins, S., Pencheon, D., Brayne, C. and Williams, R. (1994) *Dementia: Health care needs assessment: The epidemiologically based assessment reviews*, London: DoH.

Moriarty, J. (1998) 'Carers and the role of the family', in J. Pathy (ed) *Principles and practice of geriatric medicine*, 3rd edn, Chichester: John Wiley.

Moriarty, J. and Levin, E. (1998) 'Respite care in homes and hospitals', in R. Jack (ed) *Residential versus community care: The role of institutions in welfare provision*, Basingstoke: Macmillan.

Moriarty, J. and Webb, S. (1995) *An evaluation of community care arrangements for older people with dementia, First Report*, London: NISW.

Moriarty, J. and Webb, S. (1997) 'Carers' experiences of community care', *Alzheimer's Disease Society Newsletter*, October, p 7.

Moriarty, J. and Webb, S. (1998) *Charging for community care services*, London: NISW Research Unit.

Moriarty, J., Levin, E., Pahl, J. and Webb, S. (1994) *An evaluation of community care arrangements for older people with dementia*, London: NISW.

Morris, R., Morris, L. and Britton, P. (1988) 'Factors affecting the emotional wellbeing of caregivers of dementia sufferers', *British Journal of Psychiatry*, vol 153, pp 147-56.

Mozley, C., Huxley, P., Sutcliffe, C., Bagley, H., Burns, A., Challis, D. and Cordingley, L. (1999) '"Not knowing where I am doesn't mean I don't know what I like": cognitive impairment and quality of life responses in elderly people', *International Journal of Geriatric Psychiatry*, vol 14, pp 776-83.

MRC CFAS (Medical Research Council Cognitive Function and Ageing Study) and RIS (Resource Implications Study) (1999) 'Profile of disability in elderly people: estimates from a longitudinal population study', *BMJ*, vol 318, pp 1108-11.

Myers, F. and MacDonald, C. (1996) 'Power to the people? Involving users and carers in needs assessments and care planning – views from the practitioner', *Health and Social Care in the Community*, vol 4, no 2, pp 86-95.

Myers, K. and Seed, P. (1993) 'Issues arising from two contrasting life styles', in A. Chapman and M. Marshall (eds) *Dementia: New skills for social workers*, London: Jessica Kingsley.

National Health Service and Community Care Act 1990, Chapter 19, London: HMSO.

Netten, A. and Beecham, J. (1993) *Costing community care: Theory and practice*, Aldershot: Ashgate.

Netten, A. and Dennett, J. (1996) *Unit costs of health and social care*, Canterbury: Personal Social Services Research Unit.

Netten, A. and Topan, C. (1996) 'The costs of care', in J. Schneider (ed) *An exploration of the measure of quality of care*, Discussion Paper 1245, Canterbury: Personal Social Services Research Unit.

Nocon, A. and Qureshi, H. (1996) *Outcomes of community care for users and carers*, Buckingham: Open University Press.

Nolan, M. and Grant, G. (1992) *Regular respite: An evaluation of a hospital rota bed scheme for elderly people*, London: Age Concern England.

O'Connor, D., Pollitt, P., Brook, C. and Reiss, B. (1989b) 'The distribution of services to demented elderly people living in the community', *International Journal of Geriatric Psychiatry*, vol 4, pp 339-44.

O'Connor, D., Pollitt, P., Brook, C., Reiss, B. and Roth, M. (1991) 'Does early intervention reduce the number of elderly people with dementia admitted to institutions for long term care?', *BMJ*, vol 302, pp 871-5.

O'Connor, D., Pollitt, P., Roth, M., Brook, C. and Reiss, B. (1990) 'Problems reported by relatives in a community study of dementia', *British Journal of Psychiatry*, vol 156, pp 835-41.

O'Connor, D., Pollitt, P., Hyde, J., Brook, C., Reiss, B. and Roth, M. (1988) 'Do general practitioners miss dementia in elderly patients', *BMJ*, vol 297, pp 1107-10.

O'Connor, D., Pollitt, P., Hyde, J., Fellows, J., Miller, N., Brook, C., Reiss, B. and Roth, M. (1989a) 'The prevalence of dementia as measured by the Cambridge Mental Disorders of the Elderly Examination', *Acta Psychiatrica Scandanavia*, vol 79, pp 190-8.

ONS (Office for National Statistics) (1998) *Annual abstract of statistics*, London: The Stationery Office.

OPCS (Office of Population Censuses and Surveys) (1990) *Standard occupational classification*, London: HMSO.

Opit, L. and Pahl, J. (1993) 'Institutional care for elderly people: can we predict admissions?', *Research, Policy and Planning*, vol 10, no 2, pp 2-5.

Parker, G. (1990) *With due care and attention*, 2nd edn, London: Family Policy Studies Centre.

Parker, G. (1998) 'Impact of the NHS and Community Care Act on informal carers: Briefing paper for the Royal Commission on Long Term Care for the Elderly', Paper presented at the seminar 'Caring for People Five Years On: What Have We Learned About the Impact of the 1993 Act on the Care of Frail Elderly People?', Leeds.

Parker, G. and Lawton, D. (1994) *Different types of care, different types of carer*, London: HMSO.

Parry-Jones, B. and Caldock, K. (1995) 'Assessment and practice after [the] reforms: a view from the workshops', *Newsletter,* Summer 95 edn, Centre for Social Policy Research and Development, pp 13-18.

Patel N. (1999) *Black and minority ethnic elderly: Perspectives on long term care*, Research Volume 1 of the Report by The Royal Commission on Long Term Care, London: The Stationery Office.

Patel, N., Mirza, N.R., Lindblad, P., Amstrup, K. and Samaoli, O. (1998) *Dementia and minority ethnic older people: Managing care in the UK, Denmark and France*, Lyme Regis: Russell House.

Petch, A., Stalker, K., Taylor, C. and Taylor, J. (1994) *Assessment and care management pilot projects in Scotland: An overview*, Stirling: Social Work Research Centre, Community Care in Scotland Discussion Paper 3, University of Stirling.

Petch, A., Cheetham, J., Fuller, R., MacDonald, C. and Myers, F. with Hallam, A. and Knapp, M. (1996) *Delivering community care: Initial implementation of care management in Scotland*, Edinburgh: The Stationery Office.

Phillipson, C. (1992) 'Family care of the elderly in Great Britain', in J. Kosberg (ed) *Family care of the elderly: Social and cultural changes*, Beverly Hills, CA: Sage Publications.

Philp, I., McKee, K.J., Meldrum, P., Ballinger, B.R., Gilhooly, M.L.M., Gordon, D.S., Mutch, W.J. and Whittick, J.E. (1995) 'Community care for demented and non-demented elderly people: a comparison study of financial burden, service use and unmet needs in family supporters', *BMJ*, vol 310, pp 1503-6.

Philp, I., McKee, K.J., Armstrong, G.K, Ballinger, B.R., Gilhooly, M.L.M., Gordon, D.S., Mutch, W.J. and Whittick, J.E. (1997) 'Institutionalization risk amongst people with dementia supported by family carers in a Scottish city', *Aging & Mental Health*, vol 1, pp 339-45.

PPP Lifetime Care (1996) *What do they really think? Attitudes towards long term care*, Stratford-upon-Avon: PPP Lifetime Care plc.

Pushkar Gold, D., Feldman Reis, M., Markiewicz, D. and Andres, D. (1995) 'When home caregiving ends: a longitudinal study of outcomes for caregivers of relatives with dementia', *Journal of The American Geriatrics Society*, vol 43, pp 10-16.

Qureshi, H. and Walker, A. (1989) *The caring relationship*, Basingstoke: Macmillan Education.

Qureshi, H., Patmore, C., Nicholas, E. and Bamford, C. (1998) *Outcomes in community care practice, Number Five, Overview: Outcomes of social care for older people and carers*, York: Social Policy Research Unit.

Ramsay, M., Winget, C. and Higginson, I. (1995) 'Review: measures to determine the outcome of community services for people with dementia', *Age and Ageing*, vol 24, pp 73-83.

Reddy, S. and Pitt, B. (1993) 'What becomes of demented patients referred to a psychogeriatric unit? An approach to audit', *International Journal of Geriatric Psychiatry*, vol 8, pp 175-80.

Redmond, E., Rudd, A.G. and Martin, F.C. (1996) 'Older people in receipt of home help: a group with high levels of unmet health needs', *Health and Social Care in the Community*, vol 4, no 6, pp 347-52.

Riordan, J.M. and Bennett, A.V. (1998) 'An evaluation of an augmented domiciliary service to older people with dementia and their carers', *Aging and Mental Health*, vol 2, pp 137-43.

Rowlings, C. (1985) 'Practice in field care', in J. Lishman (ed) *Research highlights in social work 3: Developing services for the elderly*, 2nd edn, London: Kogan Page.

Royal Commission on Long Term Care (1999) *With respect to old age: Long term care – Rights and responsibilities*, Cm 4192-I, London: The Stationery Office.

Schaum Resau, L. (1995) 'Obtaining informed consent in Alzheimer's research', *Journal of Neuroscience Nursing*, vol 27, pp 57-60.

Schneider, J., Mann, A. and Netten, A. (1997a) 'Residential care for elderly people: an exploratory study of quality measurement', *Mental Health Research Review*, vol 4, pp 12-15.

Schneider, J., Mann, A., Mozley, C., Blizard, R., Abbey, A., Egelstaff, R., Levin, E., Kharicha, K., Netten, A., Todd, C. and Topan, C. (1997b) *Residential care for elderly people: Policy implications from an exploratory study*, Discussion Paper 1251, Canterbury: Personal Social Services Research Unit.

Secretaries of State for Health, Social Security, Wales and Scotland (1989) *Caring for people: Community care in the next decade and beyond*, Cm 849, London: HMSO.

Secretary of State for Health (1997) *The new NHS: Modern, dependable*, Cm 3807, London: The Stationery Office.

Secretary of State for Health (1998) *Modernising social services: Promoting independence, improving protection, raising standards*, Cm 4169, London: The Stationery Office.

Sheppard, M. (1995) *Care management and the new social work: A critical analysis*, London: Whiting & Birch.

Silliman, R. (1993) 'Predictors of family caregivers' physical and psychological health following hospitalization of their elders', *Journal of the Americal Geriatrics Society*, vol 41, pp 1039-46.

Simpson, R., Scothern, G. and Vincent, M. (1995) 'Survey of carer satisfaction with the quality of care delivered to in-patients suffering from dementia', *Journal of Advanced Nursing*, vol 22, pp 517-27.

Sinclair, I., Parker, R., Leat, D. and Williams, J. (1990) *The kaleidoscope of care: A review of research on welfare provision for elderly people*, London: HMSO.

SSI (1996) *Assessing older people with dementia living in the community: Practice issues for health and social services*, London: DoH.

SSI (1997) *At home with dementia: Inspection of services for older people with dementia in the community*, London: DoH.

SSI (1998a) *Care management study*, London: DoH Social Care Group.

SSI (1998b) *They look after their own, don't they? Inspection of community care services for black and ethnic minority older people*, London: DoH Social Care Group.

SSI (1999) *Meeting the challenge: Improving management information for the effective commissioning of social care services for older people*, London: DoH Social Care Group.

SSI/SWSG (Scottish Office Social Work Services Group) (1991a) *Care management and assessment: Practitioners' guide*, London: HMSO.

SSI/SWSG (1991b) *Care management and assessment: Managers' guide*, London: HMSO.

Spackman, A., Glastonbury, B. and Gilbert, D. (1997) 'There's no such thing as a simple piece of information', *New Technology in the Human Services*, vol 10, pp 10-14.

Spicker, P. and Gordon, D. with Ballinger, B., Gillies, B., McWilliam, N., Mutch, W. and Seed, P. (1997) *Planning for the needs of people with dementia: The development of a profile for use in local services*, Aldershot: Avebury.

Stalker, K., Gilliard, J. and Downs, M.G. (1999) 'Eliciting user perspectives on what works', *International Journal of Geriatric Psychiatry*, vol 14, pp 120-34.

Sturges, P. (1997) 'Dementia care management: healing the split', in M. Marshall (ed) *Dementia: State of the art*, London: Centre for Policy on Ageing, pp 123-9.

Taylor, C. (1993) *An evaluation of a multi-disciplinary pilot project 'Assessment of Social Care Needs' for elderly people in Borders Region*, Social Work Research Centre Paper 32, Stirling: University of Stirling.

Teri, I.. (1999) 'Training families to provide care: effects on people with dementia', *International Journal of Geriatric Psychiatry*, vol 14, pp 110-19.

Thornton, P. and Tozer, R. (1995) *Having a say in change: Older people and community care*, York: Joseph Rowntree Foundation.

Tinker, A. (1997) 'The other side of the fence', *BMJ*, vol 315, p 1385.

Tulle-Winton, E. (1993) 'Do you remember your social worker? Interviewing the elderly clients of social work teams', Paper given at British Society of Gerontology Annual Conference, 22nd Annual Conference, Norwich.

Twigg, J. (1988) 'Models of carers: how do social care agencies conceptualise their relationship with informal carers?', *Journal of Social Policy*, vol 18, pp 53-6.

Twigg, J. and Atkin, K. (1994) *Carers perceived: Policy and practice in informal care*, Milton Keynes: Open University Press.

Twigg, J., Atkin, K. and Perring, C. (1990) *Carers and services: A review of research*, London: HMSO.

Ungerson, C. (1987) *Policy is personal: Sex, gender and informal care*, London: Tavistock.

Vitaliano, P.P., Young, H.M. and Russo, J. (1991) 'Burden: a review of measures used among caregivers of individuals with dementia', *The Gerontologist*, vol 31, pp 67-75.

Walker, A. (1995) *Half a century of promises*, London: Counsel and Care.

Warnes, T. (1996) 'The age structure and ageing of the ethnic groups', in D. Coleman and J. Sale (eds) *Ethnicity in the 1991 Census, Volume One: Demographic characteristics of the ethnic minority populations*, London: OPCS.

Webb, A. and Wistow, G. (1986) *Planning, need and scarcity: Essays on the personal social services*, London: Allen and Unwin.

Wells, Y.D., Jorm, A.F., Jordan, F. and Lefroy, R. (1990) 'Effects on care-givers of special day care programmes for dementia sufferers', *Australian and New Zealand Journal of Psychiatry*, vol 24, pp 1-9.

Wenger, G.C. (1990) 'Elderly carers: the need for appropriate intervention', *Ageing and Society*, vol 10, pp 197-219.

Wenger, G.C. (1992) *Help in old age – Facing up to change*, Occasional Paper 5, Liverpool: Liverpool University Press.

Wenger, G.C. (1994a) *Support networks of older people*, York: Joseph Rowntree Foundation.

Wenger, G.C. (1994b) 'Support networks and dementia', *International Journal of Geriatric Psychiatry*, vol 9, pp 181-94.

West, P., Illsley, R. and Kelman, H. (1984) 'Public preferences for the care of dependency groups', *Social Science and Medicine*, vol 18, pp 287-95.

Weyerer, S. Häfner, H., Mann, A., Ames, D. and Graham, N. (1995) 'Prevalence and course of depression among elderly residential home admissions in Mannheim and Camden', *International Psychogeriatrics*, vol 7, pp 479-93.

Whitlach, C.J., Zarit, S.H. and von Eye, A. (1991) 'Efficacy of interventions with caregivers: a reanalysis', *The Gerontologist*, vol 31, pp 9-14.

Wijeratne, C. and Lovestone, S. (1996) 'A pilot study comparing psychological and physical morbidity in carers of elderly people with dementia and those with depression', *International Journal of Geriatric Psychiatry*, vol 11, pp 741-4.

Wimo, A., Ljuunggren, G. and Winblad, B. (1997)
'Costs of care and dementia care: a review',
International Journal of Geriatric Psychiatry, vol 12,
pp 841-56.

Woods, R. (1992) 'Psychological therapies and their
efficacy', *Reviews in Clinical Gerontology*, vol 2, pp
171-83.

Appendix 1: Comparisons between participants and non-participants

Table A1: Percentage of eligible referrals interviewed for the study

Situation at referral	Percentage interviewed		Percentage of refusals		Percentage of remaining non-interviews		n
Type of carer							
Spouse or daughter	63	ref	21	ref	16		98
Other relative	83	*	9	*	15		46
No carer	77	*	2	*	13		53
Social worker exclusion person from study							
Yes	74	**	14		12	***	188
No	11	ref	0		89	ref	9
SSD							
Metropolitan borough	70		14		16		94
London borough	79		6		15		34
County	70		17		14		69
All	72		13		15		197

Note: *p* values are based on logistic regressions, which use a reference category for the statistical test (marked 'ref').

*	$p < 0.05$
**	$p < 0.01$
***	$p < 0.001$

Table A2: Levels of cognitive impairment within the study population as measured by the NISW Noticeable Problems

	Mean problem score (0-6)*	n	p
Interviewed			NS
Yes	3.38	141	
No	3.81	56	
Not interviewed			NS
Refusals	3.80	27	
Other reason	3.89	170	
Location of older person at assessor interview			0.000
Community	3.3 (±0.29)	123	
Hospital, residential or nursing care	4.6 (±0.33)	74	
SSD			0.009
Metropolitan borough	3.43 (±0.35)	94	
London borough	4.26 (±0.54)	34	
County	4.10 (±0.37)	69	
Type of carer			NS
Spouse or daughter	3.80	98	
Other relative	3.95	46	
No carer	3.63	53	
All	3.78	197	

*The sample mean 95% confidence limits are shown in brackets.

Appendix 2: NISW Noticeable Problems

Does [name of person] ... have noticeable problems in:

....	Yes	No
(1) Remembering recent events?	❏	❏
(2) Working out how to do some basic everyday tasks .... such as dressing, making tea, going to the toilet?	❏	❏
(3) Knowing the time?	❏	❏
(4) Knowing where he/she is?	❏	❏
(5) Correctly naming persons seen regularly?	❏	❏
(6) Keeping in touch with a conversation?	❏	❏

© Crown Copyright 1989

Appendix 3: Summary of schedules used with informants

Separate schedules were designed for carer, proxy informants and people with dementia. They consisted of open and closed questions on different topics which were supplemented by standardised measures. Informants were invited to make any additional comments of their own. Copies of the schedules are available from the Research Unit. With the exception of the standardised measures that were not developed by NISW, for which separate permission must be sought, the full schedules or individual questions may be used with permission.

Schedules for carer and proxy informants

Sections marked with an asterisk were completed only by carers.

	Topic	Content of questions
1	Interview information	
2	Introduction	Explanation of research and request for consent to participate in study
3a*	Demographic information about the carer	Age, gender, ethnic background, employment status, type of accommodation and tenure, household composition
3b	Demographic information about the older person	Age, gender, ethnic background, employment status, type of accommodation and tenure, household composition
3	Frequency of contact with older person	*Additional questions for carers on transport and length of journey time. Visits to and from older person.
4*	Time as a carer	Length of time caring, identification of problems experienced by the older person, reactions to caring
5	Assessment	Identity of referrer, arrangements made for assessment to take place, identity of assessor and others present for assessment, content, what was offered, what actually happened, contact with assessor since assessment
6	Long-term care	Venue, cost, date of admission
7	Domiciliary and other home-based services (home care, home-based care, meals on wheels)	Provider, cost, and frequency of service; what help was provided, benefits and disadvantages to older person, problems and suggestions for improvement; if not currently using the service, whether it has been used in the past. *More detailed questions for carers, who also reported on their views of the service
8	Day care	As for 7
9	Short-stay care	As for 7
10*	Carers' groups	Whether carer has attended, whether carer would like to attend
11a	Health contacts	Frequency and content of contact with GP, old age psychiatry/healthcare of older people services, community nurses (including CPNs)
11b	Other services	Contact with other professionals, use of privately arranged services
12*	Long-term plans	Feelings about long-term care – has it been offered, would it be accepted?
13*	Carer's health	Self-rated health or limiting long-standing illness, contact with GP, GHQ-28 (Goldberg and Williams, 1988)
14*	Carer's social contact	Contact with family and friends, confiding relationships, leisure and holidays and whether they have been affected by caring
15	Support to older person	Assistance with ADLs and IADLs from carer/proxy, services, and others (eg other family members)
16	Behaviour of older person	Positive traits (warm, not critical, helpful, not demanding, cheerful, not abusive or aggressive, appreciative, interested in surroundings) and trying behaviours (clinging, repetitive actions/words, restless, non-recognition, destructive, loses/hides things, embarrassing behaviours, tearful, aggressive). *Additional questions for carers on feeling close, temper loss (Levin et al, 1989)
17*	Life events and difficulties	Life events, household tension and problems at work, income and benefit
18	Future plans	What informant thinks is likely to happen
19	Interviewer comments	

Schedule for people with dementia

	Topic	Content of questions
1	Interview information	Summary of demographic details on older person and service receipt, location of interview
2	Introduction	Explanation of research and request for consent to participate in study
3	Screening for dementia and depression, severity of dementia	Answers to a 38-item structured questionnaire (Brief Assessment Schedule, Macdonald et al, 1982) are used to produce scores for the OBS and the DEP; DEP items omitted if none of the four OBS filter questions are answered correctly
4	Assessment	Identify whether participant remembers assessment; content of assessment and participant's reaction to process
5	Home care	Identify whether participants with home care remember service; content of visits, likes and dislikes
6	Meals service	Identify whether participants with meals remember service; likes and dislikes
7	Home-based care service	As for 5
8	Day care	As for 5
9	Short-stay care	As for 5
10	Long-term care	Experiences of living in long-term care; likes and dislikes
11	Other topics	Other help; help from family and friends; past life and employment
12	Interviewer comments	